The diagnostic process

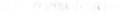

The diagnostic process

A MODEL FOR CLINICAL TEACHERS

JOHN I. BALLA

*Neurologist, Prince Henry's Hospital, Melbourne; Dean of the
Prince Henry's Hospital Clinical School
and Hon. Senior Lecturer, Monash University, Melbourne*

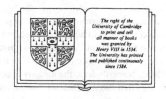

The right of the
University of Cambridge
to print and sell
all manner of books
was granted by
Henry VIII in 1534.
The University has printed
and published continuously
since 1584.

CAMBRIDGE UNIVERSITY PRESS

Cambridge

London   New York   New Rochelle

Melbourne   Sydney

CAMBRIDGE UNIVERSITY PRESS
Cambridge, New York, Melbourne, Madrid, Cape Town, Singapore, São Paulo, Delhi

Cambridge University Press
The Edinburgh Building, Cambridge CB2 8RU, UK

Published in the United States of America by Cambridge University Press, New York

www.cambridge.org
Information on this title: www.cambridge.org/9780521103572

© Cambridge University Press 1985

First published 1985
This digitally printed version 2009

A catalogue record for this publication is available from the British Library

Library of Congress Catalogue Card Number: 85–23056

ISBN 978-0-521-30213-5 hardback
ISBN 978-0-521-10357-2 paperback

CONTENTS

PREFACE

This book is offered to clinical teachers. My aim is to introduce some of the basic concepts which have recently been applied to the studies of the diagnostic process and to medical problem solving in general. The subject is important because of its implications for medical education as well as in the reassessment of clinical medicine as a scientific activity.

Most of us who combine clinical practice with teaching would have little time or expertise to analyse our activities. Yet, it has been shown repeatedly that our actions as clinicians may not coincide with our teaching (Campbell 1976). There appears to be a distinct gap between what we do and what we teach. I believe that in order to close this gap we need to research and analyse both aspects of our actions. Our task as teachers is to help students acquire an understanding of what we do. I would agree with Stenhouse (1975) that 'a teacher ... does not teach what he alone knows, letting his pupils in on secrets. On the contrary, his task is to help his pupils gain entry into a commonwealth of knowledge and skills, to hand on to them something which others already possess'.

One of the main reasons for presenting this book is therefore to make teachers more aware of the principles underlying their clinical work so that they will be in a better position to transmit knowledge to students. The numerous facts students have to learn are more likely to acquire meaning if there is a structural theory behind them (Stenhouse 1975). Similar sentiments are expressed by Dudley (1982), lamenting the lack of a clear theoretical framework relevant to clinical education.

Indeed, we are facing an incongruous situation in which students who are destined to spend their working lives gathering information from patients, making decisions and solving problems, are taught little, if anything, about the basics of information processing and of decision making. Doctors are thoroughly grounded in the so-called basic sciences such as anatomy and physiology; however, they are rarely instructed in the logic of what for most of them will constitute the bulk of their professional activities – information gathering and decision making. There are possibly several reasons for such a discrepancy. It may be thought that the methodology of the physical sciences should suffice for the methods of clinical medicine, or it may be considered that such a nebulous entity as clinical diagnosis could not be approached in a systematic scientific manner. It is likely that there are also historical reasons. When medical schools were founded, there were no scientific theories of information processing and decision making. These are largely the accompaniments of the computer explosion.

There have been recent trends to remedy this situation. A review by Elstein (1981) shows an increasing number of medical schools developing an interest in teaching the rationale of medical decision making. However, teaching is often done by non-clinical teachers and psychologists rather than by clinicians actively involved in the practice of medicine. Therefore, the relevance of this teaching, at least in the students' mind, may be divorced from clinical medicine. It would therefore seem all the more important for clinical teachers who are practising as clinicians to be well versed in the science of clinical diagnosis.

The field is rapidly enlarging and most publications have appeared over the past 10 years or so. They include the work of psychologists and educators, as well as computer scientists and medical professionals. It would therefore seem appropriate to offer a single text which may make the subject comprehensible to those who are developing an interest and find some of the concepts confusing.

My emphasis throughout has been on diagnosis. I have deliberately excluded discussion on doctor–patient relationships and on treatment. This is not to suggest that these are unimportant or that they should be regarded as separate activities. My aim has been to clarify and put forward a model of a part of our work and it will be evident that this should not in any way imply lack of concern for the way we interact with patients. Reiser (1978), looking at the effect of technological advances on the practice of medicine, also draws our attention to the prospect of distancing doctor from patient. I believe that by making our actions more explicit, we should be able to safeguard against this loss. Reiser's suggestion of doctors becoming the 'prototype of technological man' must surely alert us to the need to develop and nurture a science of clinical medicine. Accordingly, one of my main concerns has been to demonstrate the possible application of scientific principles to individual diagnosis.

There are already several excellent books available. For instance Wulff (1981a) in his book *Rational Diagnosis and Treatment* deals with some of the mathematical bases of diagnosis and clarifies much of the confusion involved in different forms of clinical labelling. Murphy in *The Logic of Medicine* (1976) describes some logical and philosophical concepts applicable to clinical medicine. Elstein, Shulman & Sprafka (1978) write from their wide experience in cognitive studies of diagnosis in *Medical Problem Solving*, and Weinstein and Fineberg (1980) give a detailed study of clinical decision analysis. Kahneman, Slovic & Tversky (1982) describe the theories which form the basis of our understanding of the cognitive processes behind decision making. This book is different in that it draws together several strands of the theory, particularly those based on information processing and decision making. The perspective presented should help teachers develop new teaching concepts and methods. The practical application of these theories should also assist undergraduate medical students to emulate the technique of the expert at an early stage and derive more enjoyment from their clinical work.

The book is written from a background of clinical medicine. The clinical examples which appear throughout the text make it apparent that it is aimed at medical teachers. I believe, however, that similar principles apply to the work of the allied health professionals who also have to make a diagnosis and then base their clinical decisions on the diagnosis. Therefore, it is hoped that by use of analogy they may find the book of some interest and that it may stimulate research in their area of expertise.

The first chapter introduces the concept of a philosophy of

science. It is then shown how the particular features of clinical work make a scientific approach difficult, but at the same time more valuable. The main section of the book deals with theories of information processing and decision making. This is partly a review of the work of other authors and wherever possible it is substantiated by the findings of my own research in this field. Most space is devoted to an analysis of decision making. This involves a certain amount of relatively elementary mathematics and logic. I must make it clear at the outset that although I believe that an understanding of rational decision making is important, I am not advocating the everyday use of mathematical concepts or that computers supplant diagnosticians. I do believe, however, that it is essential for us to know how to use these techniques for three main reasons. Firstly, a great deal of clinical work relies on the use of rules of thumb. These are satisfactory in most situations, but require regular revision and questioning of entrenched opinion. Secondly, with advances in technology we need a technique to assess the place of new developments and the obsolescence of others. Similarly, with new methods of treatment, as for instance in oncology, we need a method to deal with hitherto unknown clinical conditions. Clinical decision analysis should help in all these spheres. The final chapter, by way of a summary, illustrates how these principles may be applied in the everyday work of students and of their teachers. Wherever possible I have used clinical illustrations to demonstrate the immediate relevance of this work. It is suggested that readers may find it useful to think of similar cases from their own recent experiences.

This book is therefore offered as an introductory text to those who wish to analyse their own diagnostic methods with the hope that it will help them in their teaching and that eventually we may be able to teach some of these concepts directly to students.

The book is the result of many years of involvement in medical education and research. Over the last few years I have also tried to teach some of these ideas to students. I believe that as I gained deeper understanding of what I was trying to achieve my success has increased considerably. I appreciate the help of my colleagues, especially those at the Neurology Department at Prince Henry's

Hospital, who acted as a sounding board and helped by criticizing my ideas. Of course, the greatest help was given by students but I must also acknowledge the special help given by a few. Drs Andrew Elefanty and David Rollo made helpful suggestions after reading parts of the manuscript. Most of my original research was carried out with the help of Ann Balla who was simulated patient, research assistant and video technician. Dr Bob Iansek collaborated with many of my studies and has been instrumental in developing many new ideas. It will be evident to all readers how much I was influenced by Professor Arthur Elstein who has done so much pioneering work on medical problem solving and more recently on applying decision analytic theory to medical education. Many helpful suggestions were made by the publishers through their reviewers at different stages of the script. The arduous and most important task of editing was done by Margaret Gibson. Diane Ryan patiently retyped the multiple versions of the manuscript.

Melbourne
July 1984   John I. Balla

1
Philosophy of science

❦

The main concern of this book is to demonstrate that there is a scientific approach to diagnosis and that this may be taught to students. This emphasis on diagnosis is not for lack of concern about the other aspects of the work of clinicians, but rather because it is apparent that there is an urgent need to develop and teach a methodology of rational diagnosis. The age-old dilemma of regarding medicine as art or science is further complicated when it is suggested that it is no more than skilled applied technology. Few would debate that the so-called pre-clinical sciences such as physiology and anatomy should be classed as forms of scientific endeavour. New advances in knowledge about understanding of diseases would again be regarded as scientific developments by all but the most extreme detractors of anything medical. Our concern here, however, is with the everyday work of the clinician seeing patients and making decisions about them. The purpose of this chapter is to demonstrate how the principles of scientific methodology may be applied to the work of clinicians and how an understanding of these principles may be helpful to students.

Science and philosophy

The first problem will be to define science and also in the present context to see if a philosophy of science is relevant, because men of medicine tend to regard themselves as action oriented and thus may find the term 'philosophy' unattractive. Popper (1972) defines science as 'any attempt to solve a definite, logical and distinguishable set of problems'. His definition therefore does not confine itself to research where there is an enlargement of knowledge through new discoveries, but he includes the analysis of the procedures of everyday activities (Popper 1976). He would include amongst the aims of science a study of methods of ascertaining facts about problems with provisional attempts at solutions. The philosophy of science is concerned with the understanding of the general principles behind our way of looking at problems and with analysing them in a systematic way. It should therefore be relevant to the everyday practice of solving clinical problems. Medawar (1969) was one of the first to suggest that scientific methodology should be applied to the act of clinical diagnosis. Campbell (1976) also regarded the dichotomy between the so-called basic sciences and clinical medicine as being artificial, and thought that clinical teaching should be given recognition as a scientific method.

The old-fashioned view of science was one of inductive thinking. The observer would have to empty his mind of all preconceived notions and watch nature in action. Having collected a great deal of factual information, theories could then be formulated to explain what had been observed. This technique is frequently taught to medical students who are admonished to collect all relevant information from history taking, examination and investigations before attempting to formulate a diagnosis. This, of course, does not really occur in everyday life. It is impossible to perform any activity without some sort of preconceived notion about the situation. This is clearly the opposite of the inductive type of method that had been advocated in the past and is still being taught. It was Popper (1972) who took things even further by his method of falsification. It will be necessary to take a brief look at this because it is basic to the method of the clinician who is acting in a rational scientific manner.

Falsification

The basis of this method is that bold hypotheses are proposed and these are then exposed to severe criticisms in an attempt at falsification (Popper 1972). We do not argue from fact to theory; the intention is to start with a theory and then make an attempt to refute it. According to this line of reasoning a new idea is put up tentatively and the theory behind the idea is tested with critical methods to try to eliminate errors. If errors are present, a new tentative solution is proposed which is again put through the same process of criticism, and the process is continually renewed. This method relies on criticizing theories rather than defending them. In our efforts to falsify, we may, of course, find what appears to be confirmatory evidence for the hypothesis being tested. It is not suggested that this should be discarded, but that it needs an even more critical appraisal than the negative evidence.

Medawar (1969) regarded such a hypothetico-deductive system as one of negative feedback rather than the perhaps more plausible one of positive feedback. The feedback controls future performance according to the result already obtained. To illustrate this with a clinical example, we may be faced with a patient who has paraplegia and the first tentative hypothesis may be that it is caused by vitamin B_{12} deficiency. If the vitamin B_{12} level is normal it will show that this hypothesis is wrong. An alternative hypothesis will then be put forward, for example that the patient has a spinal cord tumour. Specialized investigations will then be performed, which show that there is no evidence for a cord tumour. This hypothesis will then be discarded and another one put forward in the hope of finding a better solution. It is apparent that there are a number of problems inherent in this method and we shall try to give brief answers to criticisms which may arise. We need to see how the first tentative hypothesis is formulated, what sort of data may be used for falsification, and what sort of precision should be reached, so that we know when to stop making attempts at further falsification.

The first hypothesis

Popper believes that there can be no unprejudiced observation and the critical phase must be preceded by some sort of dogmatic phase upon which error elimination can begin to work. Medawar also points out that the 'imagination cannot work *in vacuo*'. He suggests that the original hypothesis entering our mind would have to be plausible and that there may be some sort of internal circuitry involved in this process. It is the formation of the original hypothesis which is the creative act of scientific enquiry and which tends to defy logic. It is suggested that this creativity is beyond logical analysis. Hitting on a hypothesis is in some ways perhaps an inductive process where with intuition we generate ideas which can then be tested.

It is likely therefore that such ideas depend on our previous experience of probabilities and utilities. If a clinician knows that most headaches are related to tension, the first idea indeed may be that the headache in the patient is one of the tension variety. If the circumstances suggest that the headache could be related to a sub-dural clot because the patient was involved in an accident, he may start from that premise and eliminate the possibility of a tension-related headache. Whether this is something that could be regarded as a creative act as suggested by Medawar, or whether it is some-thing that can be analysed, will be referred to later when looking at various decision making rules used in the clinical approach.

Reliability of data

One of the main criticisms of this method is the difficulty inherent in assessing the information to be used to falsify a theory (Chalmers 1976). It is assumed that the data used for falsification will be reliable and therefore of some significance. Yet, the information may be faulty and therefore any decisions made may be false because of the nature of the information that was used. For instance, if we say that a patient does not have a paraplegia due to vitamin B_{12} deficiency because the vitamin B_{12} level is normal, we imply that we have complete confidence in the assessment of this measurement. Yet, we know that the measurement may be false or our understanding of its significance may change with increasing knowledge. Therefore, our falsification may prove to have been made on false information.

Critics of falsification theory will also argue that there is no reason to regard negative evidence as inherently more powerful than positive, confirmatory data. We accept that, in principle, this is a reasonable criticism. In most clinical situations decision making and data evaluation are not clear cut, and possession of a high degree of scepticism should prevent us from reaching hasty con-clusions. Even if, as clinicians, we are not able to behave as orthodox Popperians, we can still use the framework of falsification to check periodically on our actions.

Again, this question will be discussed further when we look at data processing and information gathering, but it must be apparent that the scientist using these methods should be aware of the importance of being able to assess data correctly.

Precision

The next problem we have to face concerns criticisms of the severity of hypothesis testing. We have to decide just how far to take the number of alternative hypotheses formed and how far to go with repeated testing. After all, according to falsificationism all hypotheses may eventually prove to be wrong. To answer this criticism, it is stressed that it is undesirable to seek precision for its own sake as it is only useful as a means to some clear and definite end. It is therefore implied that testing of hypotheses should cease at some point where there is no increase in clarity of the situation with further information.

With our previous example of paraplegia we excluded the possibility of a vitamin B_{12} deficiency and of spinal cord compression, and we may ask what other useful hypotheses could be put forward that could be tested. There are many other causes of paraplegia, but if we know that none of them would be treatable and none of them would be a utility to the patient then we may reasonably stop testing with only a tentative hypothesis being put forward and two important ones having been reasonably falsified.

Generalizations

The final problem attached to a possible scientific methodology in clinical medicine is that medical consultation is a singular event concerning decisions about individual patients, whereas the clinician will be using general knowledge about diseases and will try to apply it to an individual. According to this method of falsification, *universal statements*,in other words generalization, should be applicable to singular statements or events. If the clinician knows that vitamin B_{12} deficiency may cause paraplegia then he can test for it and apply his general knowledge of the results to an individual patient.

The probabilistic approach

We see how these views leave us as clinicians with uncertainties. To cope with them, decision theory may be applied to medical diagnosis. This will be dealt with at length later, but we will show here how its basic concepts, which take into account the subjective probability of an event occurring and the utility of outcome, are consistent with our ideas about hypothesis formation and falsification.

The probability of an event occurring is measurable and it may be an objective property of any proposition (Hesse 1974). We do not, however, generally have prior knowledge of the true outcome. We shall have some sort of subjective belief of the likely occurrence of a future event, but no absolute knowledge of it. The weather forecast may indicate rain, so we may believe that it will probably rain tomorrow. If our beliefs are rational, we should be guided by our probability assessment of the weather forecast, unless we have some other information which we assume to be more reliable. Thus, forming the hypothesis that it will rain will depend on our degree of acceptance of the forecast as evidence.

Decision theory, then, will provide us with a framework for formulating different strategies in order to prepare for rain or sunshine. If our belief in the forecast is strong, we can cancel our previously arranged outing. If we are very doubtful, we may go ahead with the arrangements. It will be apparent that to some extent what we do will also be affected by the significance of the possible alternative outcomes. If the picnic is important to us, we may take a chance and gamble on no rain. If a large amount of money is lost by not cancelling in time, we may call off the arrangements, even if the probability of rain is low, to avoid any risk of financial loss.

To put this into a clinical context and to help us refer back to our discussions of falsification, we may think of a middle-aged patient who presents with a three-week history of diarrhoea shortly after returning from a trip abroad. The initial hypothesis may suggest an enteric infection, based on our knowledge that this is a frequent occurrence under these conditions. We also know that carcinoma of the colon may present with diarrhoea in this age group and this could be an alternative hypothesis. Faecal cultures may be positive, apparently confirming the first hypothesis. If we are suspicious of such confirmatory evidence, we may consider the data to be insufficient and still require further falsification of the second hypothesis of carcinoma, particularly if we feel that missing a carcinoma may be an unacceptable risk, requiring a higher degree of precision than is provided by a positive faecal culture. Further tests, such as sigmoidoscopy and barium enema, may then be carried out to look for evidence of falsification of the alternative hypothesis. As in our vitamin B_{12}–paraplegia example, how far we go will depend on the strength of our belief in the probability of carcinoma and on our assessment of the importance of making a diagnosis.

We may face criticisms because so much of the clinician's work is probabilistic. We also know that diagnoses often have to be based on insufficient data which may at times be of questionable reliability. This can be seen as a major problem when we try and apply principles of falsifiability to our diagnostic process. Our acceptance of the probabilistic approach and our occasional reliance on data of poor quality still do not preclude us from working within the paradigm of falsifiable hypotheses. Our final hypothesis should be potentially falsifiable; if it is not, then it should be regarded as no more than a guide for action and the clinician will have to realise that it may need urgent modification in the light of new evidence.

We may therefore go along with Medawar and believe that the clinician should observe with a purpose in mind, asking directed questions with the formation of early hypotheses and going through a sequential evaluation of the evidence. He may start off his first hypothesis with an imaginative insight, but his conclusions should be based on the scientific method. Similarly, we must encourage students to formulate early and multiple diagnostic hypotheses. They must learn to ask appropriate directed questions and they must learn to be particularly careful in evaluating the validity of the information they are using to arrive at a diagnosis.

The various forms of diagnosis, only some of which are potentially falsifiable, will be the subject of the next chapter.

2
Problems of the scientific approach

🦂

Continuing the theme of the previous chapter, we now look at the unique features of clinical work which frustrate the application of the scientific method by clinicians. Students may perceive the clinical encounter as mysterious and the expert often finds it difficult to explain the relevance of scientific method to individual cases. Teachers may therefore find it helpful to classify diagnoses into three different kinds depending on which sort of systematic monitoring of the diagnostic method is feasible in each category. Similarly, diseases will be divided into three groups according to the potential for feedback in assessing the results of medical intervention.

Three kinds of diagnosis
'Common-sense' diagnosis

This is the situation where it is almost impossible to be wrong if the clinician uses 'common sense' and has some very rudimentary background knowledge of the frequency of different diseases. For instance, if a 65-year-old man suddenly develops sudden weakness on the right side of his body, then it is almost certain that he has had some form of stroke. Similarly, a 30-year-old woman who has a long history of throbbing episodic headache associated with blurring of vision and vomiting is likely to have migraine.

The patient will often have enough knowledge to make the diagnosis, and in such high probabilistic situations lay people will come to accurate conclusions. If a doctor sees 100 such cases, makes 99 correct guesses and is wrong on the hundredth case, he will retain confidence in his relative infallibility. After all, it is only human to err and to make one mistake in a hundred cases shows good clinical sense. He is likely to think that the correct diagnoses were based on the application of years of learning and on some complex, though perhaps poorly understood, reasoning. It may not be apparent that the diagnoses were founded on common-place empirical knowledge. It is also unlikely that anyone would want to analyse the causes of errors in the unusual event of a wrong diagnosis. In any case, analysis will not be amenable to a simple statistical study and therefore it will be difficult to learn from mistakes.

We may see how in this very common diagnostic class doctors may practise, and indeed apparently do well, without the application of sound logic or of scientific concepts.

The non-falsifiable diagnosis ('I say so' diagnosis)

In this category the diagnostic label will depend on somewhat loose and variable criteria that may be used to define various clinical disorders. Such labels, which at times may be referred to as syndromes, are usually accepted within the different groups of the profession. The previous example of migraine may be used here as well, in that neurologists will define migraine in a certain way. There is at this stage no way of disproving such a diagnosis and it is accepted by other members of the profession because the neurologist says it is the correct diagnosis. Similar considerations may apply to the diagnosis of epilepsy or even of angina pectoris. Although various investigations may help to define the conditions, both electroencephalographic and electrocardiographic changes may be unreliable guides to diagnosis. The situation may arise where different professional groups within medicine give different definitions. So, the patient with the same clinical features may attract different diagnostic labels depending on which group of doctors he deals with. Someone with neckache seeing an orthopaedic surgeon may be diagnosed as having degenerative arthritis causing the neckache. The same patient seeing a doctor within the field of physical medicine may receive the diagnosis of muscle strain and perhaps some nerve root irritation. If he sees a neurologist he may be regarded as being psychoneurotic, while if he sees a psychiatrist he could be labelled as having an hysterical conversion reaction. In these cases it is almost impossible to learn from one's mistakes because so much depends on the doctor's framework of reference and beliefs about the diagnostic label.

Evidential diagnosis (falsifiable)

This is the category where some independent evidence can be obtained to prove or disprove the diagnosis. A typical example is where a biopsy may confirm the presence of a tumour. Similarly, a normal vitamin B_{12} level or normal thyroid function tests may exclude the diagnosis of subacute combined degeneration of the cord, or of thyrotoxicosis. It must be noted, however, that in many cases such a diagnosis is only potentially proven or falsified by evidence which may not actually be sought.

Three kinds of disease

As we consider the disease processes that are embraced by these diagnoses, further problems arise in relation to the assessment of results of therapy. In this context we may divide diseases into three separate groups.

Self-limiting conditions

Most viral illnesses, upper respiratory tract infections, sprains to muscles and joints and many emotional problems fit into this category. We may also add the well-known placebo effect and conclude that in this group of conditions any form of treatment, provided that it had no side effects in the first place, would result in improvement.

Conditions responding to relatively non-specific therapies

There are many conditions which would respond to many forms of therapy which need not be specific for that particular disease process. For instance, a wide range of antibiotics will cover most bacterial infections. Diuretics will similarly be useful in the management of cardiac failure due to ischaemic or valvular heart disease. It has also been shown that many psychiatric conditions will respond to a variety of therapies (Malan 1973).

Kassirer & Pauker (1981) analyse what they call the 'toss-up'. There will be many clinical conditions where divergent actions will have the same outcomes. These will often be the same situations where the greatest controversy exists between different professional groups. With the aid of rational decision analysis they are able to demonstrate that the outcomes are identical irrespective of the choice made by the decision maker. The argument will then appear to be insignificant and choices clearly dependent on personal and at times irrational preferences.

Specific responses

There remain a few conditions requiring specific forms of therapy and where the course of the disease in the absence of treatment is one of predictable deterioration. Examples may include myxoedema, juvenile diabetes or a large subdural blood clot.

The problem of self-assessment

Self-limiting conditions and those responding to relatively non-specific forms of therapy are common. Because of the action orientation of the medical profession, some form of intervention is usual. Consequently relatively few diagnostic or treatment errors will become apparent. The doctor may gain increasing confidence in diagnostic and treatment methods in the absence of a reasonable basis for such confidence.

A study of chest X-ray ordering behaviour showed that physicians tended to rely on X-ray findings to diagnose pneumonia. However, as they failed to request X-rays in all patients who eventually turned out to have a diagnosis of pneumonia, their feedback on the validity of the X-rays was imperfect. This contrasted with their self-assessment and gave them an 'illusion of validity' of their diagnostic methods (Bushyhead & Christensen-Szalanski 1981). According to the physicians' criteria, the clinical indications for ordering chest X-rays were validated because of the chest X-ray findings, but they were unaware of the number of missed cases because of poor feedback.

Table 2.1 shows some further examples. Readers may find it interesting to think of instances from personal experiences.

It can be seen immediately that these findings will affect different types of medical specialities to different degrees. For instance, a surgeon dealing with abdominal emergencies will usually have clear evidence of the correctness of his diagnosis when he opens the abdomen and sees whether the appendix is inflamed or not. He therefore mainly deals with evidential, falsifiable diagnoses. His treatment is likely to have specific results. Removal of a gall stone blocking the common bile duct will result in the disappearance of the jaundice, whereas if it were allowed to remain severe complications would arise.

A psychiatrist deals with diagnoses where the definition he himself gives will determine the diagnostic label, thus being non-falsifiable. At the same time, treatment generally has a non-specific result. A general practitioner deals with 'common sense' diagnoses because he usually sees a group of well-defined, common conditions. The majority of these will be self-limiting, such as sprains and upper respiratory tract infections, or will respond to non-specific therapy.

In a survey of patients seen in general practice (National Health and Medical Research Council 1966; Moraitis 1979), it was found that eight per cent presented with psychiatric illness and 11 per cent with some form of accident. Of the latter, 57 per cent improved in a week or less. Respiratory illness was the presenting problem in 19 per cent of patients, but of these less than five per cent were diagnosed as having pneumonia, and the others had non-specific viral illnesses or upper respiratory tract infections. A further 4.2 per cent of patients had non-specific musculo-skeletal problems and another 5.1 per cent were too ill defined for any diagnostic label. Thus, a

Table 2.1. *Examples of three kinds of diagnosis and disease*

Diagnosis	Disease		
	Self-limiting	Non-specific response	Specific response
Common sense	Back sprain	Infectious diarrhoea	Some infections in epidemics
Non-falsifiable	Viral illness	Migrane	—
Falsifiable	Skin infections	Haemorrhoids	Thyrotoxicosis

large proportion of these general practice populations have self-limiting conditions which may respond to non-specific medications and where the diagnosis would rarely be falsifiable.

Another example may be quoted from a single neurological private practice (Balla 1976, unpublished observations). Of a series of 240 consecutive patients just over 65 per cent were diagnosed as having various psychoneurotic problems and only 10 per cent had a clearly demonstrable physical disease which could be labelled 'falsifiable'.

It is, therefore, not difficult to see why different groups of doctors may have divergent problems in evaluating their actions. Some of these findings could explain why practising clinicians may not adhere to scientific methods. Most will have a constant problem with a relative paucity of reliable feedback on their results. Dollery (1978) comes to similar conclusions when he suggests that doctors may find it difficult to distinguish the effect of their own interventions from those of the 'natural resilience of the human body, regression upon the mean and the placebo effect'.

Students who have acquired a large body of factual knowledge may observe some of their seniors practising apparently effective medicine without the application of logical and scientific concepts. With the advent of the new science of information processing and of decision making this state of affairs can be reappraised. The many temptations to make short cuts, inherent in the three types of diseases and the three types of diagnoses, may then be avoided.

Clinicians will need to stress the special categories of problems relevant to each individual case, so that students may learn to question the rationale of their own decision making. Teachers must recognize that they come from varying backgrounds, ranging from the general practitioner to the specialist physician, and each of them will have their specific biases depending on their area of expertise. In order to practise effectively, the expert has to make some assumptions which need not be questioned each time he meets a new patient. To the student, however, the basis of such assumptions will not be clear and the expert must explain as well as stress the pay-off and risk of working within a given framework. For instance, a general practitioner who has seen six cases of gastroenteritis over the previous week may have found that they all settled within 24 hours, simply responding to dietary change and fluid administration. On meeting a new case, he will then find it unnecessary to arrange for stool cultures or treatment with antibiotics. The student will need to see this as an exercise in probabilistic diagnosis, using common sense, there being no need to make a specific and falsifiable diagnosis. This would then set the scene for diagnostic review and questioning if the response to the relatively non-specific therapy is not as expected.

We may turn to some early studies of the 'diagnostic process' to show that the process itself can indeed be dissected and put under close scrutiny.

Some basic studies of the diagnostic process

Dudley (1968) suggested that because the diagnostic process itself was capable of investigation and analysis, it could be taught to students, thus improving their diagnostic skills. He stressed the importance of the utility of the diagnosis which he referred to as the 'pay off', and the use of heuristics, in other words goal-seeking behaviour, in arriving at this diagnosis. He also pointed out that a great deal of the diagnosis depended on pattern recognition. Kleinmuntz (1968) felt that the highly structured nature of the clinical data presented to the neurologist makes it amenable to analysis. After looking at a number of neurologists he concluded that 'clinical intuition' was conducive to 'rigorous scientific study'. Wortman (1972) also studied an expert neurologist and found that most of the questions asked by the neurologist were directed at testing specific hypotheses. He remarked that the neurologist only tended to remember what he regarded as pertinent information, forgetting the rest. Elstein *et al.* (1972) used 'actors' to study the diagnostic process of expert physicians. They showed that the process commenced with early hypothesis formation and that specific hypothesis-testing questions were asked. They pointed out that this scheme was contrary to material generally taught to medical students. In another study, de Dombal (1978) showed that the diagnostic process was subject to marked individual variation. He indicated that the expert used an efficient method, where the questioning adapted itself to the diagnostic problems, whilst the novice tended to ask stereotyped questions more or less in a clerical manner. Lustèd (1968) introduced mathematical concepts into clinical decision making whilst Salamon and colleagues (1976) applied computer technology to the study of neurological diagnostic problems. They were able to demonstrate that much of the diagnostic process could be replicated by the computer.

All of these studies indicate the apparent differences between the expert and novice, and emphasise the paradox whereby the technique of the expert is different from the teaching the expert gives the student. It therefore seems reasonable to take the analysis of the diagnostic process further and this requires knowledge and understanding of some of the basic theories which are involved in this scheme.

3
Information-processing theory
AN OVERVIEW
🍇

This chapter gives a general overview of information-processing theory and puts it into the context of the diagnostic process.

Most previous work on medical problem solving assumed the importance of information-processing theory and in this regard the work of Newell & Simon (1972) has been most influential. Their volume on *Human Problem Solving* presents a detailed model of information gathering and processing. Much has of course been written since, but their work retains its influence and their model appears the most appropriate of the theories concerning information processing.

It will be shown in this chapter how data obtained from the patient are matched with knowledge already available to the problem solver. We know that patients come to see us as doctors expecting us to solve their problems. The doctor is the problem solver (in co-operation with the patient); he must recognize what the problem is and he must set what needs to be solved as a specific goal. The information he is obtaining should be structured with this aim in mind. He must be aware of the limitations caused by difficulties in obtaining data, the limitations of problem solvers related to their stores of knowledge and the way these are available for matching up to the problem. The experienced clinician will be well versed in all this, but it may not be apparent to the student and it will be for the teacher to make the process explicit.

We may illustrate some of these points with a middle-aged woman who comes to the Casualty Department with her husband. She is anxious, tremulous and hyperactive, with rapid breathing. Within a matter of seconds a great deal of information is thus made available. Just how much is observed will be affected by the training of the observer. What it means to him will depend on his understanding of the significance of each individual piece of information, as well as any special meaning he may give to seeing all these features in combination.

The way this is translated into something meaningful is what information processing is all about. We see that this necessarily entails a number of steps. The information must be present and observed – for example, the woman is tremulous and hyperactive. This, however, is only the first step. The bits of information must mean something to us, otherwise there is no point in being aware of them. Thus, we must have learned somewhere that hyperactivity and tremulousness in a middle-aged woman could be caused by anxiety or by thyroid disease. Our pre-existing knowledge needs to be used to make inferences about the information that was observed. How we react to this information is the next step in information processing.

Information processing may therefore be seen as a gathering and translation of present data into terms referable to past experience and theoretical knowledge. A computer will be fed data cards and will then process the information. The sailor looking at the ripples on the water and the tell-tale on the mast will also be gathering information on the strength and direction of the wind. Information processing describes behaviour over time where each new act may be regarded as the function of a preceding state. This means that when a person is seen to be performing some sort of activity, it will be a reaction to something that had occurred earlier. When we see the sailor moving the rudder and pulling in his sheets it will be a reaction to the information he gathered by looking at the water and the tell-tale. The doctor taking the woman's pulse is responding to his observations of hyperactivity and tremulousness. When we think of information processing we have to assume that the system which is performing the task must be sufficient for that particular activity. The sailor would need to have sufficient knowledge about interpreting the ripples on the water and the direction of the tell-tale to know which way to turn his boat; otherwise, even if the information is available, he will not be able to make useful decisions. Similarly, the doctor must know that a rapid pulse rate may be a sign of thyroid disease in his tremulous patient.

We know that any new discipline develops its own language so that communication between workers in the field is made easier. This has the immediate effect of making it more difficult for those who are outsiders to comprehend what a particular subject may be all about. Therefore, our first task will be to define some terms commonly used when describing information-processing systems. After this outline more details will be given on individual variables and we shall then be able to say how we may apply these concepts to our own work on the diagnostic process.

Problems

Patients generally go to see their doctors because they have a problem. This may be a headache, an irregular heart beat or loss of weight. Diagnosis follows from identifying the problem and attempting to solve it. Identification may vary in complexity from recognizing a viral sore throat simply by looking, to understanding the psychopathology in the background of a child brought by his parents for nocturnal bed-wetting.

Information processing will deal with *problems*. A problem is defined as a difficult question which requires an answer, but which an individual cannot solve because he does not know what series of actions is required. The experienced general practitioner with a good background knowledge of the family may immediately recognize the problem of the bed-wetting child and he may also be able to take steps to solve the problem. Looking at the expert meeting old situations may not tell us much because all he will do is reach for the old and well-tried solution. New situations, however, allow us to see what sort of techniques are required to identify and solve problems. The patient who comes along complaining of general fatigue may have serious organic disease or mild reactive depression. The method of sorting through the multitude of possible diagnoses is to be our concern here.

When confronted with a problem the individual will have to decide how to solve it and what sort of strategies he should be employing. Later, we will need to see what makes a problem a difficult one as opposed to one with an easy solution. Is something easy because the solution presents itself simply by looking, as the sore throat example, or is it simple because we have met the problem before, as in the case of the bed wetter? Are problems difficult because the alternatives are multiple? We shall deal with these questions in this book, because if we understand why a problem is simple or complex, we should be able to impart some of this understanding to our students.

Goal

One of the basic assumptions of information-processing theory is that human behaviour is both *goal orientated* and *rational.* An elderly patient presenting with rectal bleeding may have haemorrhoids, with one important alternative being bowel cancer. The goal of diagnostic activity must be to exclude cancer and to this end tests would include sigmoidoscopy and barium studies. The same symptom of rectal bleeding may have a different significance in someone with a known bleeding tendency or taking anticoagulant drugs. The first line of tests will then be aimed at assessing the blood-clotting factors. Similarly, a bed-wetting child with suspected family problems suggests the need to have other members of the family interviewed, rather than to have his kidneys X-rayed. A *goal* is regarded as something that a diagnostic system is aiming at and has to attain before it will be satisfied, and as something that will structure the problem-solving activity. We may take the example of a patient presenting with brief transient episodes of aphasia. We shall listen with particular care to the neck, assess his general suitability for surgery and arrange for carotid angiograms, hoping to find a surgically treatable stenotic lesion. The same symptoms presenting in a patient adamantly opposed to surgery or who had severe cardiac disease contra-indicating surgery will elicit a different course of action. Now we may concentrate our diagnostic efforts in assessing the advisability of anticoagulant therapy or aspirin. If there is a suspicion of an active peptic ulcer, tests may need to include gastroscopy whilst this would have been of little concern in the first example where we were thinking in terms of cerebral angiography. Given the same initial situation with different goals, differently structured problems will arise. The patient with rectal bleeding may have bowel X-rays or blood tests. The bed-wetting child may have his urine tested or the psychodynamics of his family may be explored.

If we accept the assumption that behaviour is goal orientated and rational, we must see that the clinician's actions will to a large extent depend on the task in hand. With the initial symptom of aphasia, we may recommend carotid angiograms or gastroscopy depending on our intention to prepare the patient for surgery or anticoagulants.

Rational behaviour

When we say that *rational* behaviour is assumed, we imply sensible behaviour that is derived from reasoning. As we well know, human behaviour is not always rational. The errors inherent in information processing were demonstrated by Simon (1957). The human mind needs to reduce complex problems to simple ones. The simplification is achieved by using rules of thumb which deal with most situations but at the same time introduce systematic errors leading to bias. These were described by Tversky & Kahneman (1974) and we shall deal with them at greater length when we discuss decision making. For the time being we should bear in mind that clinicians and students are prone to make similar errors in the use of intuitive logic and that we shall need to find some means of dealing with these errors (Balla 1980b; Borak & Veilleux 1982). There are a number of other variables which will be affected by limitations of the *problem solver* and we shall outline these now.

The process

A young woman may complain of symptoms in her hands and a burning pain waking her in the early hours of the morning. These symptoms may be regarded as the input and the problem solver, the doctor, will have some internal representation of painful hands in young women. He will attempt to diagnose the cause of the pain in the hands and solve the problem. To do this, he will need to know that the symptom of burning hands through the night is characteristic of a carpal tunnel syndrome. The goal will be to make a diagnosis, to choose a likely explanation for the pain. Treatment may then be instituted and if this fails the situation reassessed. He may then need to gather more information relevant to the original diagnosis of a carpal tunnel syndrome. For instance, nerve conduction studies may be ordered.

In a schematic way we can see information processing as consisting of inputs which are in some way translated into a symbolic internal representation within the problem solver. This will have to fit the problem so that the correct method may be selected. A particular goal must be chosen and specific problem-solving methods will follow.

In this context, a few more terms need to be defined.

The *task environment*. This is the presentation of the problem as discussed earlier. One of the basic tenets of information processing theory is that it is largely the task which will determine the method of problem solving. Rectal bleeding, bed wetting, painful hands may, as we saw, all elicit different reactions on the part of the problem solver.

Internal representation of the outside task. This may vary according to individual and speciality. We may refer to the example of the neurologist who is able to translate the symptoms of the patient into anatomical diagrams in his mind. Then, on seeing a patient with a combination of cerebellar ataxia, upper motor neurone signs and nystagmus, he may immediately visualize the relevant anatomy of the brain stem.

Problem space

The actual problem-solving activity is assumed to occur in what is called a *problem space*. This is defined as the internal space in the individual where problem solving occurs. It is an internal representation of the relevant part of the environment which is important for achieving the goal which has been set. This problem space should not be regarded as an anatomical site or a clear physiological function. Rather, it should be seen in a psychological sense and no more than a diagrammatic representation and structuring of what is happening. Here we assume that there is some sort of interface between the problem and the method that is being used to solve it. The individual must 'interpret' the situation in such a way that he is able to use his resources for solving the problem. The hyperactive, tremulous woman will bring forth in the problem solver all his past knowledge of how to deal with thyroid disease or an anxiety state.

Information sources

For this interpretation there must be information sources which can be used through the process. The sources will be coming partly from the outside environment and partly from the resources of the problem solver. These resources will relate to various memories, in other words knowledge of past situations, and the solver's technical ability to solve problems. Previous knowledge may be used for predicting the relative promises of different sorts of actions and in evaluating the efficacy of past actions. A bed-wetting child well known to his family doctor may elicit the immediate response of looking for school stress, whereas in another child the same symptoms may indicate that sibling rivalry could be the problem. If these avenues do not bring in further information, then others need to be explored, for instance the urine could be tested for infection.

Before we see what sort of methods may be useful for problem solving we must look at a particular component within the problem space: the various *memories* which are available to the information-processing system. It is customary to deal with them in three separate categories: long-term memory, short-term memory and external memory.

Memories

Long-term memory

It is often assumed that this has an infinite capacity. It may be associative so that one memory stimulus may evoke another one. Recognisable stimulus patterns give what is called a 'chunk', which may develop through learning so that we are able to associate one stimulus with another. The actual size of the stimulus may be variable and again up to a point may be a learned pattern. The experienced clinician may know that hyperactivity and tremulousness can be symptoms of thyroid disease. Upon seeing such symptoms in his patient, he may also 'remember' that they may be associated with a rapid pulse and protruding eyes.

In long-term memory is laid down what we could call *encyc-*

lopaedic knowledge. This involves all the memory traces that the individual collects through his life. A great deal of pioneering work on this subject was done by de Groot (1965), a master of chess and a psychologist. He looked at the thinking processes of chess masters and also compared them with novice players. His work is relevant to our discussion because the master with his immense experience and rapid response to the state of play on the board is comparable to the expert clinician who is able to make a rapid and accurate assessment of his patient. As a result of de Groot's work much of the literature on the diagnostic process and on problem solving is studded with chess analogies.

It was de Groot who pointed out that to be useful, knowledge must be available. This can be achieved by keeping it in a dynamic state so that any significant stimulus will make this knowledge readily available to the information processor. In terms of de Groot's original work, it is not much use memorizing the various opening moves of a game, if we are not capable of immediately associating them with the various responses that can be made. It is likely that after experience of repeated events patterns are laid down so that each new situation will evoke memories of relevant knowledge. Rectal bleeding will immediately bring to mind all the relevant facts about bowel cancer and how it is differentiated from haemorrhoids.

It is also likely that learning in an associative way will be useful in this respect. If we learn from a book the ten causes of rectal bleeding and then a week or two later we are faced with an actual patient with this symptom, it may be difficult to use the knowledge which was laid down earlier. Previous work suggests that learning the problem-solving process in conjunction with laying down the new knowledge which is essential for solving such problems may hasten the development of usable encyclopaedic knowledge. Thus, associating textbook knowledge with patients seen in the wards will help the retention of readily usable knowledge.

Short-term memory

This refers to the memory traces which are being laid down throughout the processing of information when the data are collected. Decay is rapid, often over seconds or minutes. This built-in constraint on processing the immediately available information constitutes one of the major invariables of the human information-processing system. It is here that many errors in the structuring of data will occur. It implies that only a few data can be processed at the same time.

The most significant contribution in this field was made by Miller (1956), his work having a profound effect on our understanding of cognitive psychology. He referred to 'the magic number seven, plus or minus two', drawing our attention to an important limiting factor in information processing. His original work, done with psychology students, demonstrated that they could only retain a limited amount of information and that if too much was presented to them at the same time they were unable to cope with the excess data. More recent work suggests that our limitations may be even greater, with only 5 ± 2 chunks retained. The size of the chunk may be variable and is of fairly limited length. Work on physicists and others by Simon (1974) has suggested that the size may increase with experience with a particular task. We may also think of our earlier example of the expert chess player who is able to absorb more information on looking at the board than his inexperienced opponent. It is likely that with experience people will be able to remember more associations and find it easier to deal with additional relevant factors at the same time. One may also think of the experienced clinician who has no difficulty in remembering details of a complicated history presented by the patient, whereas his inexperienced colleague will need to make constant reference to his notes. It is the situation where the senior clinician whose memory is supposed to be failing him will often outshine inexperienced youth.

It may at times be difficult to separate the effects of the limitation imposed by short-term memory span and those due to limitations in *channel capacity* (Miller 1956). Only a limited number of problems can be tackled at the same time and if the system is expected to deal with more than its built-in capacity, distraction will occur and information processing is likely to break down.

These limitations of short-term memory and channel capacity

have significant implications for information processing. They suggest that the system can easily be overloaded with too much information. An individual will only be able to deal with so many facts at once. Any other information will become redundant and as a result, if data are not carefully selected, valuable information will be lost and some unimportant features may be retained. Many readers will have had the experience of asking for directions on how to get to a certain street. If given a few details about two or three turns and perhaps one or two landmarks, the street will probably be found without too much difficulty. If the informer gives too much information about minor side streets and unimportant landscapes then it is unlikely that it will all be remembered and the enquirer is much more likely to get lost. The patient who says too much, meandering through a complex story, will also confuse us. We shall say more about this later.

External memory

Originally this term may have been applied to computer systems, but equally it could be applicable to the human information processor. Examples may include paper and pencil when doing mental arithmetic, a chess board when playing chess, writing notes while taking a history. With the use of such aids short-term memory may be significantly enlarged and thus more useful information can be processed at the same time.

The method of problem solving

We saw how information from the task environment enters into the problem space of the individual and is interpreted so that goal-oriented behaviour may take place. It is now left for us to see what sort of methods may be used by individuals to solve problems and achieve goals once the problem is recognized, understood and aligned with a goal. We saw how there must be some dynamic knowledge available which can be extracted from long-term memory and how this may be aided by external memory. We must also assume that there will be individual differences depending on the psychology, intellect and experience of the individual. All the same, there are problem-solving mechanisms which will be available to cover most contingencies. The ultimate aim of information processing is to translate the information into a form where suitable decisions can be made so that correct solutions may be reached. More will be said about decision making in the chapters on decision theory, but at this stage we could say that there are probably three main problem-solving methods in use:

1. *Hypothesis generation and testing.* This was mentioned in the chapter on the philosophy of science and it is apparent how this method would be suitable for information processing. From early clues a hypothesis is generated, and then further data are collected in order to test the hypothesis which could then be modified. The agitated woman may have thyroid disease. Her pulse is taken with the expectation that it should be rapid. If it is slow, the original hypothesis may be modified.

2. *The heuristic search.* This is a goal-oriented method and to be able to use it one must understand the structure of the problem and know the likely outcomes. Information gathering will then be oriented in such a way that the data can be used to reach the chosen goal. To this end, certain 'rules of thumb' will be used. It is a technique frequently employed by experts when dealing with familiar problems. For instance, increasingly severe headaches may be due to a brain tumour. A CT scan therefore will be arranged with the specific aim of excluding this possibility. If it is normal, the diagnosis will to all intents and purposes be eliminated.

3. *The recognition method.* This involves the reduction of a difficult problem to something that is known and recognized. Exactly what is recognized in coming to useful decisions is something we shall deal with later. It can be said now that this is the sort of situation where the answer is immediately obvious to the experienced observer so that he is able to make an immediate translation of the problem into a solution. A crushing central chest pain coming on with exertion in a middle-aged male is recognized as being cardiac in origin.

Summary

In summary we may put the different components of information processing into the context of the diagnostic process.

Task environment. The patient provides all the outside data which will be used to process information in order to come to a diagnostic decision. How the actual data will be transmitted from the patient to the clinician is the important variable here and will be discussed in the chapter on 'Data gathering'.

The problem solver. The transmission of data has certain predetermined invariable properties which affect the way the problem solver can handle information. In particular, the limitation of the various types of memory and channel capacity concerns us here. This will be discussed in Chapter 5.

Decision making. We shall then come to see how decisions will be made about the data through the various stages of the diagnostic process. This will be discussed in Chapters 6–8.

Individual differences. Such differences between various systems may affect the outcome. In the case of clinicians this will refer to differences in intelligence, psychological and social make-up as well as degree of expertise. These problems will rate a brief mention in Chapter 9.

4
Data gathering

Following on from our general overview, in this chapter we take a closer look at the first stage of information processing and emphasize the problems inherent in gathering data from patients. The concepts of data reliability and validity will be introduced. The expert will intuitively judge information according to these criteria, but it will be a complex labyrinth for the novice. It will therefore be necessary to explain to students that judgment may be prone to error either due to problems inherent in data, the source of which is the patient, or in the problem solver. The significance of the information should be weighted in terms of specificity and sensitivity. The three sources of data, history, examination and special tests, also have their peculiar strengths and shortcomings, often taken for granted by the expert but not generally recognized by the student.

We start with an example of a 50-year-old woman complaining of a recent onset of stiffness in her right hand. She had difficulty in fine manipulations, such as using cutlery, doing up her buttons and her handwriting had become small. Blood tests for rheumatoid arthritis were negative, as were X-rays of her wrist, and nerve conduction studies were also normal. Examination by another doctor revealed that she had paucity of fine movement and cogwheel rigidity, both characteristic of Parkinsonism. On being informed that she had Parkinson's disease she had difficulty comprehending how this could be the case when she had previously been told that all her tests were normal. She queried why she was told that the tests were satisfactory, when according to her understanding they obviously could not have been normal. The situation that had to be made clear to her was that the tests were indeed normal, but that they were done for an irrelevant condition. She did not need tests for arthritis: she needed tests for Parkinson's disease. The tests were good and reliable, but they had no significance, no *validity* in her situation.

Another case in point concerns a 65-year-old man who complained of backache and weight loss. His doctor, suspecting serious pathology in his lumbar spine, ordered a plain X-ray and later a CT scan to exclude secondary cancer. Both of these tests were reported as being normal. The patient was then told that there was nothing seriously wrong and that he should just rest to get over his muscle strain. When the pain became more severe he went to see another doctor who arranged for tests on the assumption that the previous ones were normal. Eventually, when the original X-rays were reviewed, the diagnosis of secondary cancer deposits was made. In this case, the tests ordered were indeed relevant and of high validity, but too much reliance was placed on the radiologist who reported the film. The information was therefore of poor *reliability*. These two cases illustrate some of the crucial problems inherent in the first stage of information processing which is data gathering. This evaluation process is an essential step before the information can be used for problem solving. It is not enough to obtain the data: it will also be necessary to judge it in the context in which it will be used.

Judgment consists of putting the data on a sliding scale before attempting to draw inferences from it. Any piece of information may be judged as being good, indifferent, or poor. The report on the spinal X-ray was judged as being reliable, and the tests on a woman with Parkinsonism were judged as relevant. It would not be very difficult for the experienced clinician to think of other examples within his own area of expertise. A frequently heard question on ward round is: 'Who reported on it?', when we discuss an X-ray or a pathology report. This implies that we had made an assessment of the reliability of our radiologist or pathologist and will place more or less reliance on the report, depending on this judgment. Similarly, on hearing that our patient with headache or shortness of breath has an abnormal calcium level, we may ask the intern why the test was ordered and how it will affect the management of our patient. These may be extreme, though common enough, examples to emphasize that experienced clinicians are well aware of the problems we are discussing but that their junior colleagues need frequent reminders.

We may see how this discussion is relevant to the pursuit of the scientific methodology which is based on falsification as its major premise. If the data which are to be used for falsifying a hypothesis are unreliable, or of little significance, such as the X-rays and nerve conduction tests in our original examples, then any conclusions drawn must necessarily be invalid. That is why it is so important to understand how data are to be judged.

As correct data evaluation is one of the hallmarks of expertise, it will be useful to know what kinds of systematic *errors* may occur when making judgments. We may see two possibilities: the clinician may overvalue data, or alternatively underrate what was good evidence. In the case of nerve conduction studies we may conclude that our patient has no significant physical illness when the finding was irrelevant. In the case of the pathology report we may not accept the findings when they were in fact accurate and relevant.

Stewart, Joyce & Lindell (1975) analyse the two kinds of error which may occur, drawing an analogy with the two types of error of the null hypothesis of statistical inference. Good information may be rejected and, as with Type I errors of the null hypothesis, this would imply lack of confidence in the data. Alternatively, poor information may not be rejected, leading to results equivalent to the Type II error of the null hypothesis when we fail to reject a false hypothesis. This would imply insufficient care with the examination of our data. In the first instance our criteria for acceptance were too high, in the second they were too low. The latter is a common problem affecting students. It will be necessary for students to be aware of the features of the data which may result in faulty judgment. As shown by de Dombal (1978), the two aspects of medical data that will need careful attention will be the reliability and the weighting of information.

The first of these, the *reliability* of the data, may be affected by observer error. Inter-observer reliability refers to the degree to which doctors will agree with each other's findings, whilst intra-observer reliability refers to the degree to which the same judge's assessments can be reproduced. If two observers disagree on the size of the heart in a patient then this will be regarded as inter-observer unreliability. If the same observer on repeated examinations comes up with the same measurement of cardiac size then one may say that there was no intra-observer variation and his assessment was reliable. It does not, however, indicate that the measurement was accurate because the heart size measured by some other, and perhaps better, method, may be shown to be much larger than originally assessed. An extensive review of the reliability of medical data (Koran 1975) demonstrated the existence of unreliability in all three spheres of history, examination and special tests. Even with blood pressure measurements unreliability may be demonstrated (Hedley & Pearson 1981) and there may be significant variations depending on the degree of expertise. The implication of all this is that students must be reminded that they will need to understand their own limitations in assessing data they obtain and that they will also need to know what sort of reliability they may expect from their teachers. It should be understood that some data are inherently more reliable than others so that, for instance, a systolic murmur at the apex will be reliably assessed even by the inexperienced but a mid-diastolic rumble or fourth heart sound will be a much more unreliable sign even amongst experts. It will be important in teaching to emphasize reliable data because unreliable information so often will be associated with faulty judgment. This aspect of clinical features is frequently ignored when we teach students, yet it is good practice to impress on them that they should base judgment on reliable data. If a diagnosis depends on the interpretation of a dubious shadow on a chest radiograph we would be very hesitant to place too much reliance on it, in contrast to the appearance of recent finger clubbing, a history of excess weight loss or bronchscopic findings.

Next, we look at the *significance* of the information we have obtained. We must see what sort of weight we should be attaching to it when making decisions about the diagnosis. Certain bits of information will have more significance than others. For instance, we may know that an extensor plantar response will always indicate that a patient has a disturbance of his cortico-spinal pathway. To complicate matters, however, this piece of information has to be seen in the context of the situation which is being assessed. This means that the actual importance of a particular piece of information will depend on the circumstances. The extensor plantar response may indicate that the patient has a cortico-spinal disturbance, but it may be quite irrelevant to the problem in hand if his main complaint was shortness of breath after exertion. This is what we mean by the *validity* of our data. Our observation of the plantar response does not have any effect on our assessment of the shortness of breath in our patient. In the same way we eventually come to ignore the results of rheumatoid tests in the woman with the stiff hand. This is a most important point to bear in mind when choosing what to observe and when interpreting the significance of our observations.

More will be said about the correct weighting of information in the chapter on decision making, but two terms, specificity and sensitivity, will be introduced here (Griner *et al.* 1981). The *specificity* of a finding is a reflection of how often someone with a particular disease in the population under study will have a truly negative finding for that test. Put in different words, it indicates absence in non-diseased persons and therefore refers to the degree of certainty that a positive outcome will give in establishing the presence of a diagnosis. Such data will therefore be useful in *confirming* a suspected diagnosis. For instance, if we regard investigation *A* as being highly specific for determining the presence of disease *X*, then we can say that if investigation *A* is positive we may be reasonably confident that disease *X* is present. A glucose tolerance test is a specific test for diabetes, and if it is abnormal we shall be reasonably confident that our patient does have diabetes. Glycosuria is relatively non-specific, in that there are many conditions apart from diabetes which will be associated with the presence of glucose in the urine. Conversely, *sensitivity* is a reflection of how often we shall have a truly positive test result in the presence of disease. Under these circumstances, if an investigation results in negative findings, we may have some degree of certainty that a particular disease has been excluded. This is useful in *ruling out* a diagnostic possibility. For instance, if investigation *B* is very highly sensitive to the presence of disease *Y*, then we could say that if investigation *B* is negative we may be reasonably certain that disease *Y* will be absent. If investigation *B* is positive, then it would imply that disease *Y* may or may not be present, but we cannot give this any degree of accuracy because that will depend on specificity. A fasting blood glucose is a sensitive test for diabetes and if it is normal we may be confident in excluding most cases of diabetes.

In order to give more accurate answers we need to know not only the specificity and sensitivity of our findings, but also how often the disease is present in our population. A discussion on this will be deferred to the chapters on decision making. It must be stressed that for effective information processing, students will need to be taught the correct weights of the data they will be using. Instead of learning lists of clinical features of diseases, they will have to learn the actual significance of each of these elements in relation to each other.

We may now look at the three data sources in a little more detail. Amongst many clinicians there was at one stage a trend towards accepting investigations as being the most useful form of data for clinical decisions. There is, however, an increasing awareness of the importance of history as opposed to examination findings and investigations in coming to a diagnosis. In one reported series (Hampton *et al.* 1975) 66 of 80 diagnoses were made on history alone, examination findings contributed to seven and laboratory investigations to a further seven diagnoses. There is no doubt that this will vary in different circumstances; for example listening to a cardiac murmur may give a great deal of information which may not be obtained from taking an accurate history. On the other hand, talking to a patient who describes the evolution of his neurological symptoms is more likely to give a pathological diagnosis than any examination findings. In the two cases cited at the beginning of the chapter, the diagnosis of Parkinson's disease would be made on history and physical examination findings, whereas in the second patient with secondary cancer deposits special tests are particularly important. The point to stress is that all three aspects of the data source have to be evaluated and the one which is the cheapest, at least from the patient's point of view, history taking, needs to be looked at with the greatest care. The aim of the following survey is to make readers aware of the various pitfalls inherent in data gathering. It is hoped that after reading through these readers may analyse their own processes so that eventually they will recognize the problems encountered by students.

Data from history
Reliability

Patient error. Medical data may be affected by their source, the patient. Data coming from an inanimate object, such as the computer, cannot unknowingly be manipulated and any error in interpretation is therefore dependent on the observer. When information comes from a patient, the situation is different; he first has to interpret his sensations himself and then pass these on to an outside observer. Thus, the opportunity for errors in interpretation is increased tremendously (Havens 1978).

There are many patients who struggle when they try to explain to others what they are feeling. Even if they understand it themselves, they have *difficulty communicating it in words*. They may not understand what the doctor is trying to find out from them. An example is the case of an intelligent accountant who was complaining of episodes of instability. He expressed this as feeling giddy. His doctor asked him to explain what he meant by being giddy. It is well known that some patients will refer to blurring of vision or a full feeling in the head as well as a floating sensation under this term, whereas others may only describe themselves as being giddy when there is an actual sense of instability and maybe of rotation. Therefore, a clear understanding of what the patient means can be very important. This particular man could not understand why anyone would have difficulty in comprehending what he meant by being giddy and it took many questions and repeated misunderstandings before it became apparent that to him it did indeed imply a sense of instability.

There will be other situations where the patient does not have sufficient verbal ability or sensitivity to describe his feelings in words and cannot go beyond saying that he feels unwell and that he has a pain somewhere. Under such circumstances, the doctor who is the observer could be in an impossible situation because he would not be able to assess to his own satisfaction what the patient is trying to tell him. The expert will usually know when to stop and change the direction of his enquiry. Students with their lack of experience will find this difficult and may spend a great deal of time trying to obtain information which will not be forthcoming.

Timing of events is very important in most diagnostic situations, yet it is well known how unreliable memory may be when we come to assess this aspect of the symptomatology. We often see a situation where at the beginning of history-taking a patient says a particular symptom has been present for weeks and yet towards the end he is talking in terms of years.

There will be patients who tend to *deny* their symptoms either for some sort of psychological reason or there may be cases of patients purposely misleading the doctor. This is frequently noted when patients are asked about drug intake, alcohol or smoking. This is not an infrequent problem when litigation is pending, and people purposely give misleading information.

There remain many other unexplained problems perhaps related to poor memory, poor understanding of past events or of the questions being asked by the doctor. One study quotes nearly 35 per cent of patients who gave the wrong information about a history of circumcision and 15 per cent of mothers who were inaccurate about important details of labour which had taken place only four hours earlier (Komaroff 1979).

There is no doubt then that many patients are rightly described as 'difficult'. How can we overcome all these problems? The first thing we have to do is *recognize* when the history is likely to be unreliable. Just how this is done is something that we do not quite understand to this date. The expert should be good at this, but teaching it to students is not easy. Our criteria may be vague, but we become suspicious when meeting a patient who contradicts himself during history taking, or when the patient's manner appears to be evasive. The statements of patients who are intellectually affected, when there is obvious evidence of dementia for example, should be regarded with suspicion. Incongruous statements are also significant, such as when complaints are made which do not in a common-sense way fit in with the rest of the history and examination findings. For instance, if a patient says that he has had weakness in the legs for a matter of a week or so and if he also gives a story of tripping over for months and not being able to run as a child, we would regard the information as inconsistent and thus unreliable.

Observer error. Accurate history-taking is by car the most difficult part of the diagnostic process. This is where so many errors occur and the major problem seems to be *lack of data clarification* (Balla & Iansek 1979). By this we mean that when a patient is giving his account of his problems, the observer will not clarify in his own mind just what the patient is trying to tell him. As we said earlier, this is not infrequently due to the problems the patient experiences in communicating his thoughts. Equally, the fault may lie on the side of the doctor who either has not taken enough trouble to try to understand what is going on, or does not have enough knowledge to understand what the patient is trying to tell him so that he is unable to put symptoms in their proper categories. This lack of clarification of the data is one of the major problems of novice students. Most experienced observers on hearing a particular symptom will ask leading questions to try to clarify the picture. In contrast, we find students writing down the statements given by the patient without a clear understanding of what he is trying to communicate. A patient complaining of diarrhoea will have to be asked a number of questions to define what he means. He may indicate no more than two or three well-formed stools a day in contrast to someone who has watery and blood-stained motions every couple of days. The two types of symptoms would have different implications and unless the terms given by the patient were completely clarified, they would be useless for information processing.

Weighting of evidence

Most textbooks give lists of symptoms and of physical signs which may be found in particular diseases. Such a list will be of limited usefulness when assessing the data, because it is important to know the significance of the presence *or* absence of clinical features. In other words, the evidence must be weighted according to its importance. The situation is further complicated because the importance of particular symptoms may vary depending on what other symptoms are present in the individual patient.

We may take the example of chest pain. It is known that cardiac pain is usually centrally situated, crushing or dull and may radiate up towards the neck and left upper limb. All these bits of information are irrelevant in comparison with the actual timing of the pain. By far the most significant evidence in favour of diagnosing cardiac pain would be its relationship to exertion and relief by rest. Therefore, a person who is concentrating on a description of the quality and associated features of the pain and at the same time ignores precipitating factors may arrive at the wrong conclusion. He may miss the information that the pain was related to postural change suggesting that it was not cardiac, or that it was always related to exertion and relieved by rest, diagnostic of heart disease.

Similarly, we may look at a patient who complains of facial pain and we suspect trigeminal neuralgia. We know that this is always within the strict anatomical boundaries of the fifth cranial nerve. Therefore, a description of the anatomical site of the pain will be crucial. As soon as the patient says that the pain radiates into his neck, we know that he does not have trigeminal neuralgia, as it is now outside the trigeminal distribution. Then, the associated features, such as sharp, severe episodic pain brought on by eating, will assume a new significance and suggest that it is likely to be toothache.

Unfortunately, relatively little has been done about formally quantifying the usefulness of data of this nature. We shall discuss this further when dealing with decision making in a later chapter.

Data from examination
Reliability

Reliability with physical examination is only achieved by repeated practice and constant self-criticism. It is very easy for a doctor to assume that the data he is collecting from the physical examination will be reliable and, therefore, may be used as hard factual information. It takes a great deal of honesty for an expert to admit that although he may be good at eliciting the plantar response, he may be second rate at assessing heart sounds. There is a large individual variation within the so-called normal range which adds to these difficulties. For students, it will be better to try and concentrate on

learning some basic important physical techniques rather than trying to find out about unusual signs with questionable reliability.
The first responsibility of students will be to learn the normal range,
a difficult task in a teaching hospital where one is surrounded by
unusual pathology and exposed to the temptation of learning every-
thing about abnormality and little about the normal. For instance,
there are very many ways of eliciting the plantar response apart
from stroking the sole of the foot. Each has an eponymous name
attached to it, and one sees students eagerly learning all these techniques and trying to interpret them. Yet, the expert knows how difficult it is to assess even the simple basic Babinsky-type response. It
is much better then, to try to concentrate on teaching one or two
important techniques, rather than learning many different kinds
which will be difficult to assess accurately. Any uncertainty of our
own reliability should also be taken into account when coming to
the next stage which is the weighting of the information obtained.

Weighting of examination findings

Students may find it difficult to understand that examination findings should, wherever possible, be used to check on the data
obtained from the history. The information from the history should
generate certain hypotheses as discussed earlier. The data provided
by the examination should then be used to see if there is any confirmation of the hypothesis, or if new data may lead to a revision of
the original hypothesis. What is even more important is to understand that if the examination findings are completely contrary to the
expected, it may be necessary to revise the history or check on the
reliability of the examination.

For instance, if the patient is complaining of weakness in his legs,
it may be related to an upper or lower motor neurone lesion. In the
case of the first, we would expect upper motor neurone signs with
brisk reflexes and an extensor plantar response. In the case of a
lower motor neurone lesion, flaccidity with absent reflexes would
be seen. The examination findings will then confirm one or other
hypothesis. To carry this a little further, though, if the history indicated that the patient had his symptoms for a matter of three weeks
only, then gross wasting or marked spasticity with flexion

deformities would make us realize that the history could not possibly be correct. The patient will then have to be questioned again to see if he can give a better account of time sequence. Again, in a patient who denies a history of any alcoholic intake, examination findings of liver palms, spider naevi and firm irregular liver would raise doubts about the reliability of the original history.

As we saw with the data from the history, data from examination findings can be weighted according to the situation. For instance, an extensor plantar response will always imply an upper motor neurone lesion, though brisk reflexes need not. This is well recognized by experts who work in the field, but is often forgotten by students who are not taught the importance of so-called pathognomonic features of particular conditions.

Another illustration of the changing significance of data comes from a patient who is only able to give a vague history of the onset of some weakness on the right side. Examination may be difficult, but may suggest that there is indeed some questionable weakness on the right. It may turn out then that the visual field examination shows a clear-cut field defect also to the right. The rather vague history and, up to this stage, vague examination findings would all fit in with what seems to be a definite abnormality, all making sense and supporting the diagnosis of a left hemisphere lesion. The visual field loss on the right side will, therefore, be heavily weighted evidence in the case of this patient.

Data from investigations
Reliability

It is amazing how often special investigations are regarded as being absolutely reliable by the general public, doctors and students alike. Yet, it is in this field that observer error has been best demonstrated on many occasions. Comparison of relatively simple procedures such as reading of electrocardiograms or of straight-forward chest X-rays shows large individual variation. One must assume that in some of the newer techniques observer error is also likely to be high, especially at a stage when expertise is lacking. Some tests are inherently difficult to interpret and therefore will always have a certain amount of observer error no matter what the level of expertise.

For instance, it is known that vertebral angiograms are much more difficult to interpret than angiograms in the carotid territory. Any conclusions drawn from them must therefore be regarded with some degree of suspicion. What is probably more important is the variation between observers. With electro-encephalograms and even plain chest X-rays, for instance, there will be those who 'over read' as opposed to those who 'under read' the evidence. This means that some observers will report on findings that others will tend to ignore. Before ordering a test the clinician should try to note what level of expertise and reliability to expect from his colleagues.

Weighting of information

As with physical examination findings, special investigations should be regarded as an extension of hypothesis testing. The data collected should therefore be used to confirm or refute hypotheses previously generated. To do this effectively the student will need to have a clear understanding of the specificity and sensitivity of the various tests he is using and he must know just why the tests were ordered, to exclude or to confirm a hypothesis.

For instance, a patient who has blackouts may have cardiac monitoring. If during an actual blackout the electrocardiogram shows a complete block, we shall say that this is a specific finding for a Stokes–Adams attack. Specificity in this instance should be 100 per cent. At the same time, we also know that many patients may be monitored without recording an episode so that the sensitivity of the test, monitoring, may be no more than 30 per cent. This would therefore be a good test for confirming a hypothesis, but it would have little weight as a test of exclusion. A different situation may arise when a cervical myelogram will show abnormalities with bony indentations in a 40-year-old patient. Since it is known that such changes are common in that age group, the finding of indentations in a patient with paraparesis would be a relatively non-specific change with accuracy of no more than, say, 30 per cent. On the other hand, a normal myelogram in such a patient would be a relatively sensitive indicator, say 90 per cent, that he does not have cord compression related to cervical spondylosis. Therefore, this would be a useful test of exclusion of cord compression if we understand the limitations imposed by possible non-specific features of the data.

Having reviewed some of the problems inherent in data gathering, we may now turn to see what sort of natural constraints the system will be working under.

5

Limitations on data handling

This section pays particular attention to the way the diagnostic process is affected by the inherent limitations on data handling. We have so far been discussing some problems of medical data collection and we know that the variations in information processing are largely dependent on the task in hand. At the same time there are natural constraints built into information processing systems, in this case the clinicians. Therefore, data will need to be structured in such a way that clinicians should be able to cope with processing them in a satisfactory manner. Students will frequently experience difficulties with data collection because they will not be aware of their limitations as data processors. As a result, even if they possessed the necessary encyclopaedic knowledge, it is possible that they could not use this knowledge in the appropriate clinical situation. Even if they collect the 'right' information, they may gather too many data, so that they will find it impossible to sort through all the available evidence. This may be seen in the copious notes taken by some students when they write up case histories. Some of these excesses will be due to a lack of knowing the difference between significant and insignificant information. Equally, there will be a lack of understanding that the mind cannot handle too much information at once. An understanding of these 'given' limitations should help to develop a sensible structuring of information. We shall start our discussion with reference to the storage of the encyclopaedic knowledge which is required for clinical work.

Long-term memory

In most medical schools, students spend the first two or three years of their training acquiring large stores of information, mainly about anatomy, physiology and pathology. Then, throughout his career the practising doctor has to absorb a great deal more factual information from journals, books and meetings so that he is expected to 'keep up to date'. The main problem will be to store this knowledge in a dynamic state to make it readily available at the required time.

Anyone who has experience with medical teaching will realize that there are considerable gaps in the students' ability to access information. To explore this, medical students were studied within six months of finishing their anatomy examinations. The results showed a marked discrepancy between anatomical knowledge and an ability to associate this with relevant symptoms and physical signs (Balla 1980*b*). Many had forgotten the details of anatomy even in the few months since their examinations. Those who did remember relevant facts found it impossible to apply and associate them with the appropriate clinical problems. This was in contrast to a group of expert neurologists who were able to associate their anatomical knowledge with the clinical situation. One answer to this discrepancy may be that the experts had used this information repeatedly and therefore only had to reach out for old recipes. There are suggestions that human memory works in an associative way and that it may be more useful to store information in such a way that retrieval will be facilitated. It is manifest that textbook knowledge does not equal past experience in terms of problem-solving ability.

We may well ask if there are any particular aspects of *textbook knowledge* that are making it difficult for students to assimilate the data in a usable and readily available form. We would want to see if there is any way in which the structuring of the information may not be optimal when presented to the inexperienced novice.

One obvious answer may be that some data are simply not available, and can only be accumulated through long personal experience. This would apply to the weighting of certain cues, such as the nature of the pain in coronary artery disease or the frequency of multiple joint involvement in rheumatic fever. It is only over the last few years that systematic data collections have been published such as de Dombal's (1978) work on abdominal pain.

A close look at some modern textbooks will lead us to other possible answers. For instance, a recent British textbook of medicine

(Macleod 1977) lists numerous symptoms associated with migraine, without giving any clear indications of the specificity or sensitivity of symptoms beyond terms such as 'in general', 'more worrying', 'often' and so on. There is almost no mention of negative features which could be used to rule out the condition. An equally popular and influential American text (Wintrobe *et al.* 1980) lists over 20 positive features of migraine, but no negative information. For the clinical diagnosis of angine pectoris, over 30 positive characteristics appear, in contrast to one negative feature. The same influential book, when discussing the differentiation of migraine from cerebral tumour states that it may be 'necessary to resort to a complete neurologic survey' and then lists multiple investigations as well as physical examination.

It must be evident that such large compendia of positive information, with almost complete lack of negative statements, indicate that medicine, as described in modern texts, is not based on the scientific mode. Rather, the emphasis on positive data demonstrates that the old-fashioned inductive method is advocated. The lack of negative information is consistent with the lack of any attempts to view diagnosis as being potentially falsifiable. Is it any surprise then that students spend their time searching for more and more information, instead of using the scientific method of looking at a few pieces of evidence which may then be used to substantiate or disprove an hypothesis? A different emphasis in textbook knowledge may help the learning process by reducing one of the major causes of diagnostic errors made by students, emphasis on gathering the wrong sort of information and not learning to evaluate what is significant.

It is not easy to learn long lists of information without a clearly defined structure. The knowledge students possess will have no obvious and direct relevance to how medicine is to be practised in actual life. This lack of the apparent continuity of the experience, and the lack of clear integration of practice and textbook learning is contrary to the basic educational principles as enunciated by Dewey (1963). He speaks of the 'experiential continuum' and believes that it is essential to organize and structure subject matter so as to fit in with the learner's pre-existing experiences and real life usage. The absence of these main features will explain many of the difficulties inherent in the use and retention of much textbook knowledge in long-term memory.

Short-term memory and channel-capacity limitations

Students have a lack of understanding of these natural constraints, which causes serious problems when they try to structure data. We are well aware of the brief, but relevant, history taken by many experts in complete contrast to the large amount of data collected by most students. The latter will often be sidetracked and will not remember to deal only with the important facts. This, of course, is partly due to lack of knowledge as to what is relevant. If students are taught how to weight information correctly, they may be in a better position to make the best of these built-in limitations. We also know that the expert is able to memorize larger chunks of information than the novice. For instance, we may see a neurologist who on finding an extensor plantar response, and knowing that this is frequently associated with increased tone and reflexes in the limbs, will have little difficulty in regarding this as a single chunk of information. The inexperienced student, who is not so clearly aware of this association, may have to treat each of these pieces of information separately, thus limiting his capacity to remember.

When we come to channel capacity we may speculate that it is here that the so-called *problem-oriented approach* to medical data collection may be useful. If we are able to subdivide the problems of the patient into separate categories, and then deal with them one or two at a time, it should be easier to process information. We all know about patients who are described as their own worst enemies. Some are unable to limit themselves to giving a relevant account of their symptoms and if the doctor receives too many data, even about the same problem, he will find it impossible to focus his attention correctly. Some are unable to keep to the point and will mix up their various problems, again making it more difficult for the clinician to sort out each problem separately.

The *ordering of the data* presents further difficulties. This can create major problems for students. Most specialist clinicians will collect information in a sequence which is in keeping with their specialized framework. A patient with indigestion seeing a psychiatrist will have to give a full psycho-social history as a first step. The same patient seeing a gastroenterologist will first have to describe how his symptoms relate to meal times. Students tend to order their questioning according to their most recent experiences and as a result come to disparate conclusions, depending on the orientation of their last group of teachers. This is in keeping with the increasing evidence which suggests that the order in which the information is presented will affect information-processing activity. Following the observation that clinicians had a tendency to ignore late information, we studied physicians using case vignettes where the most significant diagnostic cue was presented either at the end, or at the beginning of the sketch (Balla 1982). There was a significant difference in the diagnoses reached, in that when the cue was given late, it was ignored more often than when it was given early. This would suggest that clinicians may have difficulty in using late cues once they have a great deal of positive information contrary to the significant information which reached them 'too late'. In another study, using computer simulation techniques, Fox (1980) demonstrated that the order of cue presentation affected the choice of diagnostic alternatives. When knowledge about one disease, tonsillitis, was made available before cues about another one, laryngitis, then tonsillitis was diagnosed more often than in the latter case. It is concluded that 'the earlier something comes to mind, the greater its chances of influencing the subsequent chain of thought'.

Therefore, we may presume that we can only process information adequately if the data are structured in such a way that only a limited amount of information has to be processed at the same time. Efforts must be made to collect the most critical information early. In an ideal situation, the patient will present the history, describing his various symptoms. He may perhaps complain of a combination of headache, vertigo and double vision. This will give a brief overview of the situation comparable to the stage of *orientation* described by de Groot (1965) when the chess player looks at the board. Following this brief and spontaneous account, the initial data may be treated sequentially. The relevant information may give cues so that suitable hypotheses can be formed. For instance, the complaint of headache may make us think of the diagnosis of migraine as the first hypothesis. Further questioning will be aimed at finding data to support or reject this tentative solution. Similarly, early hypotheses may be formed about the other complaints which can then be followed up separately, and it may also be seen whether or not they can all be fitted into a single problem.

How the actual decisions on data acceptance and rejection will be made and when it will be decided to stop data collection in this process, is something we shall discuss when we look at decision making in the following chapter. The essential thing to recognize here is the need to structure data in relatively small groups so that sequential processing can be performed within the limitations of the system that is available.

External memory

This concept of computer science has some interesting implications when we study information processing as applied to medical work. It is apparent that doctors use external aids regularly to assist their memory and information-processing capacities. It is customary to write notes while taking a history and, in a less obvious way, looking at a patient may also 'nudge' our memory. After one study on the diagnostic process in which neurologists and students were videotaped while taking a history, many were surprised to see how much time they had spent writing notes, not looking at the patient but concentrating on the paper in front of them instead (Balla & Iansek 1979). Some were upset and felt that this would result in loss of rapport. There have been a number of studies to show that when clinicians do not take notes, but spend more time looking at the patient, they may gain some points, but will lose a great deal of factual information.

Apart from such immediate external aids, there will be many others which will influence data collection and decision making. A library within easy reach for reference or a recently qualified registrar will be excellent sources of up-to-date information.

Internal representation

The example of the neurologist with the readily available and well-developed internal representation of anatomical structures was given earlier. It is likely that a better understanding of how information is perceived would help in the learning process and this is another sphere where the findings of educational psychology may be usefully applied to developing new teaching methods.

Gale's (1980) work supports earlier studies suggesting that for knowledge to be useful it must be in an accessible, dynamic state. This knowledge consists of 'content', referring to factual knowledge about diseases, and 'process', whereby this factual knowledge may be used and applied in specific clinical situations. Clinical information obtained from the patient is incorporated into the structure which is perceived as being relevant to the data. From the structure 'extrapolations' are made; in other words, inferences occur. The sort of inference that will be made will depend on assessing which piece of available information has the most 'forceful features'. These forceful features are regarded as important evidence which can be used and attached to relevant structures. The assessment of what is a forceful feature will clearly depend on pre-existing knowledge and it would appear that evidence requires a certain amount of weight before it will be of sufficient value to allow a diagnostic formulation to be made.

Having seen how information will be collected at the various stages of the diagnostic process, how this may be stored and how it may be represented in the clinician's mind, we shall now turn to see how decisions will be made along the diagnostic pathway.

6

Decision making

INTRODUCTION

☙

In the following chapters we shall discuss the next stage of the diagnostic process – decision making. Most clinicians would believe that a 'good' history and examination are the main pre-requisites of a 'good' diagnosis. It is assumed that if we obtain accurate data, we shall arrive at the right conclusions. This implies that given the same information, different clinicians will make similar decisions. As has been shown repeatedly, this is not the case. Experienced physicians given identical data will come to diverse conclusions (Balla *et al.* 1983). It is at this decision-making stage of the diagnostic process that the most fundamental errors will occur and senior clinicians are essentially just as prone to these as their juniors (Berwick, Fineberg & Weinstein 1981). It will therefore be necessary for clinical teachers to be well versed in the theories of decision making applied to diagnosis.

Decision making means that we have to make choices between alternatives (Payne 1973). The aim is to make a choice which will be associated with a probability of increased utility and decreased risk of error to the decision maker. When we say that an alternative choice is associated with a certain *probability*, we mean that the outcome is uncertain and all we can aim for is that our choice will have a reasonable likelihood of being the right one. When we say that we hope to reduce the *risk* of making an error, again we mean simply that we are hoping to eliminate bad choices as much as possible. We hope that the choice which will be made will be useful to the decision maker, that it will be the most advantageous outcome of the available alternatives and that it will have a certain amount of *utility*.

A patient with Hodgkin's disease in clinical remission may develop backache and sciatic pain. Before we decide on the treatment to offer him we need to know whether nerve root compression is caused by a disc protrusion or a lymphomatous deposit. Decision strategies may then be developed to deal with various outcomes in this probabilistic environment. We shall follow different paths depending on our degree of belief in the parameters of clinical remission and on our assessment of the radiological findings or the character of the pain. A *decision strategy* may then be defined as a set of general instructions for each possible outcome in a given choice situation (Hesse 1974). In another clinical context, if a jaundiced patient suspected of having alcoholic liver disease has a liver scan which is suggestive of secondary deposits, our diagnostic hypotheses will be affected by our degree of belief in the scan and in our assessment of the importance of the clinical criteria we use for diagnosing alcoholic liver disease versus secondary cancer deposits. What we do will then also be affected by our belief in the importance of treating and investigating secondary deposits or alcoholic liver disease. Decision strategies will make explicit our belief in the value of the scan, clinical assessment and the various modes of treatment.

Decision theory. A systematic study of how choices are made in an uncertain environment, decision theory involves the investigation of various properties of differing decision strategies and is able to take into account an assessment of the decision maker's utilities as well as his belief in probabilities. It provides a framework for representing choice problems in association with utility and probability assessments (Wulff 1981*b*). Two models of decision making may be developed within this framework, normative and descriptive (Slovic, Fischoff & Lichtenstein 1977). The first, *normative theory*, deals with the mathematics and logic of decision making. It concerns itself with the actions of idealized 'statistical man' (Peterson & Beach 1967) whom we assume to be making correct choices based on logical thinking and statistical theory. He will be an optimal model for making decisions under conditions of uncertainty. The second, *descriptive theory*, systematizes the rules whereby choices are made in real-life situations. It describes the activities of men involved in decision making in specific situations.

Most empirical work on decision making demonstrates significant differences between the models of normative and descriptive
decision makers (Kahneman & Tversky 1973). As we mentioned in
the introduction to this book, such differences are important;
decision makers 'get away' with their errors and biases because our
environment is structured in such a way that many errors remain
hidden, and we have relatively little reliable feedback (Slovic *et al.*
1977).

We need to compare the working of statistical man with the
activities of his real-life brethren to see if there are any systematic
discrepancies between the two. In the following pages we shall
mention normative theory as it applies to the work of a clinician and
we shall then concentrate on describing decision models applied to
realistic problems, demonstrating how systematic bias may occur
and how this could be detrimental to optimal decision making.
Before doing this, however, we must turn to one of the most basic
concepts of decision making, the assessment of utility.

Utility

By saying that we make the best, or most suitable choice, we are
implying that it will have the highest utility as perceived by the
decision maker. It will be regarded as the most attractive of the
available choices and that is why it will be preferred to all other
alternatives.

Whilst at first sight the concept of utility may appear to be a
simple one, on a closer look it becomes one of the most difficult subjects to define and quantify. A utility consists of assigning a value to
a possible outcome (Weinstein & Fineberg 1980). To complicate
matters, not only are the attitudes of people to the desirability of
events unstable through time (Fischoff, Slovic & Lichtenstein
1980), but clear preferences may be lacking, especially when faced
with unfamiliar situations. To grasp the concept of these shifting
attitudes, we need to do no more than look at the way voters' preferences change over the last few weeks before an election. If the issues
are not clear cut, there will be a large number of 'undecided' preferences, all those people who cannot perceive the 'utility' of one
candidate over another. We may, therefore, well understand how in

a completely unfamiliar, emotionally laden situation, such as an illness, the assignment of values to the desired end may be impossible. After all, how can a value be assigned to something that is not understood.

In order to overcome some of these problems, Weinstein & Fineberg (1980) suggest the method of *utility analysis*. This involves putting utilities on a scale, so that the higher the value, the greater the utility, and the more preferred will be that outcome. Conversely, a poor outcome, or disutility, will have a low value. For instance, we may perceive death as the worst outcome, perfectly good health as the highest utility, and grades of utilities between these two extremes. If we accept that our aim is to gain the highest value, the best outcome, then we can see how utility considerations must guide decision making and clinical strategies.

The most problematical aspect of utility measurements is the subjective nature of all such values. This is how we arrive at the concept of *subjective expected utility*. this means that when we speak of utility, we understand this to be a subjective expectation of the decision maker. A further dilemma arises when doctors have to make choices based on their subjective assessments, and these at times may well be contrary to the values of the patient. There will be situations where the patient finds it difficult to make a reasonable assessment, lacking useful knowledge of the possible outcomes, or a clear understanding of the many variables involved. Ideally, the patient should be acquainted with all the facts and participate in decision making. This is often impossible and then the doctor will have to make the decisions, based on his subjective assessment of what he regards as the greatest utility to the patient. Patients' utility assessments, however, will not only show individual variation, but will also be affected by the kind of risk involved.

Eraker & Sox (1981) studied ambulant outpatients to assess their preferences when given the hypothetical alternatives of drugs with varying therapeutic and adverse effects. They found that risk taking depended on whether possible outcomes were favourable or not. For instance, most patients risked an unlikely but severe side effect in order to have a high chance of no adverse reaction. In contrast, most would choose an intermediate therapeutic effect rather than an equal chance of either a favourable or no effect.

To illustrate just how problematical 'real-life' utility assessments are, the following example is given to show how such an analysis may be carried out. A middle-aged woman accountant developed loss of vision to the left side. A CT brain scan showed that this was due to a malignant tumour. The symptoms cleared rapidly after the administration of steroids. She was informed of the probable nature of the tumour and that it required surgery to confirm the diagnosis by biopsy, at which time partial removal might be attempted. She was also told that following this she would probably require X-ray therapy. It was explained to her that surgery involved a risk, probably close to 50 per cent, of producing some loss of visual field, but that in the absence of attempted treatment, she would be certain in any case to have the same symptoms within a matter of six months. By prolonged delay the chance of useful surgical intervention and X-ray therapy would be significantly reduced. She had difficulty in making up her mind, but at the same time wanted to make the decision herself. Utility analysis was carried out as she was obviously sophisticated with figures and in full possession of her higher faculties. She was told that if the risk of surgery were non-existent, she would obviously choose it without hesitation. If the risk were 100 per cent she would clearly refuse. What figure then, would she find acceptable? She came to the conclusion that she would take a 30 per cent chance and said 'my immediate life and well-being is worth much more to me than the uncertainty of what happens six months away'. She attached a high importance to the immediate future and regarded the 50 per cent risk of visual loss as an unreasonable gamble. It appears then that this analysis fulfilled its function and both the patient and the doctor could rest assured that the correct decision was made to postpone surgery. Yet, within days, she returned after having sought multiple, mainly lay opinions, and found it impossible to accept that her personal utility assessment was the correct one. There was clearly far too much emotional investment and she doubted her own ability to make a rational choice.

This example illustrates how what appears to be a rational, subjective utility assessment may still leave the participants in doubt and confusion. Most patients still tend to 'leave it to the doctor' who will then have to make a responsible decision, trying to understand what his patient would want and what would be the best utility under the circumstances; an impossible task which will need to be tackled by the medical profession if it is to retain powers of decision making.

Many doctors are aware of these problems, even if they have trouble dealing with them. We know that utility considerations enter all phases of the diagnostic process, from the formation of the initial hypothesis, to the choice of complex investigations. To illustrate this point, a study by Pilowsky & Durbridge (1979) showed that what they called diagnostic perfectionism differed a great deal from one disease to another. Conditions where definitive and useful treatments were available would have a high utility for making a correct diagnosis. In other conditions where a positive diagnosis may imply a poor prognosis, the need for high diagnostic accuracy is important as a false positive would have very significant implications for that patient. At the other extreme, in situations where no reasonable treatment was available and where the condition had little effect on life, diagnostic utility would be low and accuracy would be relatively unimportant.

As part of another study on the diagnostic process (Balla *et al.* 1983), expert gastroenterologists were asked to rate the diagnostic significance of a number of different diseases. Only one of 27 experts said that he could not see how this would be done; in general there was high agreement in the assessment of the significance and utility in diagnosing various disease categories. For instance, the diagnosis of carcinoma of the colon is generally rated very high, but that of irritable colon is often rated low, especially amongst surgeons. Interspeciality differences were apparent in such studies and will affect patient management which may depend on what sort of specialist opinions are sought.

Clinical decision making may be divided into two stages. The first is the stage of *evaluation*. This is concerned with looking at the data to assess when sufficient information has been accumulated for decision making. The second stage will be one of making a *choice* between competing hypotheses and eventually accepting the final one. The two stages of evaluation and of choice are of course interdependent. We shall now look at some rational models and see how they may be applied to clinical work.

7
Decision making
RATIONAL MODELS

꩜

Many clinicians will abhor the idea that uncertainty may creep into medical decision making. They may say that one must not make decisions about life with any degree of uncertainty; we cannot take gambles and risks with our patients' health and we must not play games with computers or with symbolic logic when it comes to the lives of human beings. However, when we speak of decision making as we do here, we will have made the basic assumption that our information sources may be incomplete or incorrect and we are indeed facing uncertainty. Therefore, mathematical models will be important and we do need some understanding of them to reach our decisions. We would agree with George Bernard Shaw (1946) and try to avoid the situation where a doctor 'draws disastrous conclusions from his clinical experience because he has no conception of scientific method, and believes . . . that the handling of evidence and statistics need no expertness'.

To try to remain brief, we shall make reference to only five rational models that cover most situations where decisions have to be made through the diagnostic process. These are symbolic logic, the Bayesean approach, gambles, the weighting of cues and decision trees.

Symbolic logic

The so-called new mathematics of medicine is not all that new, but the realization that logical concepts and mathematical ideas may be applied to medical diagnosis is relatively recent and still tends to meet with a certain amount of resistance from those who lay claim to the 'art' of diagnosis. Here, we shall give a brief outline only of how concepts of symbolic logic may be relevant to the diagnostic process. Venn diagrams and set theory, which may be seen as following on from these ideas, will not be discussed.

The basis of symbolic logic is that certain ideas, events or attributes of physical entities may be represented in a purely symbolic manner by various letter of the alphabet (Ledley & Lusted 1959; Murphy 1976). This will enable us to give a more precise definition of concepts and represent logical processes more clearly. We may denote the patient's physical signs, symptoms and diseases in this way. For instance, we may say that if a patient had jaundice, it could be symbolized with the letter X. If he has dark urine we may symbolize it with the letter Y. By convention, if there is a bar on top of the capital letter then the patient will not have that particular attribute. Thus, $\bar{X}$ means that the patient does not have jaundice, and similarly $\bar{Y}$ means that the patient does not have dark urine. If we put a full stop between the X and Y, it means that the patient has both attributes and if we put a plus sign between the X and Y, as shown here: $X + Y$, it will mean that he has X or Y or both, meaning that he has jaundice or dark urine or both of them together. Finally, a horizontal arrow means that if the patient has the attribute to the left of the arrow he will also have the attribute to the right. Thus, we may say that $X \rightarrow Y$ means that if the patient has jaundice he will have dark urine. Some may find this unnecessary as it complicates what would appear to be straight-forward thinking and common sense. Yet, it does add a certain amount of rigorous surveillance to our decision making. We may be able to show where errors are made and demonstrate them with increased clarity. In this manner, we are able to show the great difficulty experienced by many observers in dealing with negative attributes. Most people will have relatively little trouble dealing with positive findings, but in the diagnostic process, negative information is at times even more important.

On the assumption that expert clinicians use logical methods in their diagnostic work, we studied the elementary thinking process of students and experts (Balla 1980*b*). We hoped that this would throw some light on the decision-making processes and highlight the difficulties in learning rational diagnosis. Students and expert subjects were given a description of two diseases X and Y. It was stated that one symptom was never present in disease X whilst another symptom was always present in both X and Y. Three patients were described with various symptoms and the first patient had all the symptoms including the one which could never be present in disease X.

The first section could be seen as a test whether subjects would be able to see the significance of a positive distinguishing feature. In terms of symbolic logic, one could say that if criterion A is present, then condition X cannot exist: $A \rightarrow \bar{X}$. The second section was seen as a test of the statement: $\bar{B} \rightarrow \bar{X} + \bar{Y}$. In other words, if a certain symptom (attribute) B is absent then the disease X or Y cannot be present since all people with disease X or Y must have this particular symptom B. This requires an ability to think in negative terms, which is well known to be difficult for most people.

The results showed clearly that few of the subjects had any difficulty with the positive logical problem. There was a consistently low score when negative problems were involved.

Again, with the aid of symbolic logic we should be able to demonstrate how the concepts of specificity or 'pathognomonic features' and of sensitivity of clinical attributes are important and how they are assessed by different subjects. We used an example where in the presence of a certain attribute D, condition X would always be present. This could be indicated in terms of symbolic logic as: $D \rightarrow X$. It is known that people are generally good at this type of thinking. When the test was applied to students, they gave poor results and we could assume that this indicated lack of sufficient knowledge about the significance of this positive attribute.

The question was then taken further, so that a number of attributes were described as together giving rise to condition X thus, $A \cdot B \cdot C \cdot D \rightarrow X$. It was also known that attributes $A \cdot B \cdot C$ may or may not be associated with condition X so that the equation may be expressed as $A \cdot B \cdot C \rightarrow X + \bar{X}$. In spite of this, most subjects still tended to see the combination $A \cdot B \cdot C \cdot D$ as more important than just the presence of specific attribute D. We may see how this kind of exercise could help us in checking the diagnostic process and in finding where errors in the learning stages may occur. Contrary to the original hypothesis, the generally poor results from the tests in the study indicate that doctors do not use logical concepts when making a diagnosis and we could suggest that even if in the long run such methods are not essential for the expert, knowledge of this type of symbolic logic may help students to check their own decisions and even to question the methods of some of their teachers.

The Bayesean approach

This is concerned with probability revision. Most work on medical decision making assumes that Bayes' theorem is fundamental to our understanding of the diagnostic process (Beach 1975; Salamon *et al.* 1976; Wulff 1981*a*). We know that clinicians do not use this scheme, but it is a useful model for their decision making. *Bayes' theorem* looks at probability as the measure of subjective belief in the likely occurrence of events (Hesse 1974). It takes initial probability explicitly into account and revises probability in the light of new probabilistic evidence (Wulff 1981*b*). The general proposition put forward in Bayes' theorem is that our belief about the likely occurrence of a specific event will be determined by the combination of what we know about the problem in general, and what we know about the individual case in particular. From previous knowledge we shall have certain ideas about the likelihood that certain events will occur. This is what we refer to as the initial probability. The theorem allows us to take into account new data obtained about the specific situation. This new probabilistic evidence, then, allows us to revise our initial assessment of probabilities and we can estimate our new belief in the likely occurrence of an event.

We may wish to guess the sex of an unknown medical student. There would be the prior information that in that particular medical school 50 per cent of students were males. This would be insufficient information on which to make a reasonable guess. Then, on being informed that the same student wears a skirt, the new information would allow a reasonably accurate guess about the student's sex. Similarly, if we see a patient who has a cough, stuffy nose and runny eyes, we may think that he has a common cold. If we are told that the rest of the family had similar symptoms we would feel pretty comfortable with our diagnosis. If on the other hand we were informed that he had the same symptoms each time he was exposed to a certain pollen, we would change our diagnosis and suggest that he had an allergic reaction.

The statistically relevant information when dealing with Bayes' theorem may be summarized under the three headings of *prior probability*, *specific information* and *expected accuracy of predictions* (Komaroff 1979). We shall take these points in turn, before considering other aspects of the Bayesean approach.

Prior probability

This summarizes what we know about the problem before we have any specific information regarding the individual case. The probability may be referred to as *unconditional*. It will not depend on any other factors. We should know that paraplegia in a young person is most likely to be related to multiple sclerosis and that episodic weekend headaches are caused by migraine. Haemoptysis in developing countries may make us think of tuberculosis whereas in the Western world we are more likely to suggest bronchitis. Going back to the previous example about the sex of medical students, one may see how changing conditions may affect this prior probability. In 1900 most students were males; by 1950 the ratio would have been about two to three males to one female; whereas by 1980 females outnumbered males in some schools. This illustrates how a knowledge of changing local conditions may be important at the time the data are being collected and assessed. In 1900, it would have been easy to make a guess about the sex of an unknown medical student, but it becomes impossible today without additional information. Paraplegia in a young person makes us think of multiple sclerosis , but if we find that the patient spent all his life living near the equator, we would reassess the diagnosis because we know that multiple sclerosis rarely occurs there.

For a clinician, this prior probability may be regarded as a summary of his previous knowledge and experience about the significance of a particular symptom. Lack of such knowledge, a problem often faced by students, will not allow an adequate perspective of the situation. In a purely probabilistic sense, if patients were assumed to be chosen at random from a given population, prior probability of a symptom for the patient would be the same as the symptom prevalence in the population (Weinstein & Fineberg 1980). (We may define prevalence as the frequency of the symptom in the population of interest at a given time.) Clinicians, however, are not generally interested in the whole population, and their patients are not selected at random. Doctors come to categorize their patients as being in certain groups depending on some characteristics other than just the prevalence in the population at large. Such specific patient characteristics tend to involve age, sex and social class, which are combined with prevalence to constitute a revised prior probability with respect to any subsequent information. This prior probability may be seen as a reflection of the proportion of patients with certain similar characteristics.

When we read the medical literature, or listen to doctors discussing their patients, we are left in little doubt about the importance attached to the age and sex of a patient. It is likely then that experienced clinicians come to regard their data on age, sex and prevalence as a single unit and treat it as a chunk of information.

One study with case vignettes where age and sex were used as cues suggested that experienced physicians tended to use this information as a single chunk, which the novice was less likely to do (Balla 1982). In spite of this, even experienced clinicians will frequently ignore rates of disease prevalence, which results in diagnostic errors (Balla, Elstein & Gates 1983).

Specific information

This refers to the data that we collect about the situation we are studying and which may in turn affect the likelihood of our original guess being right or wrong. On looking at our patient with the weekend headaches, we find that he has papilloedema and extensor plantar responses. We will then revise our original thoughts and feel that he is more likely to have a brain tumour than migraine.

We are dealing with individual clinical features when we assess our new information. Most textbooks teach us about disease processes and what type of clinical abnormalities may be expected with different types of pathology. Patients, however, do not come along with diseases: they come along with some sort of clinical abnormality such as headache or haemoptysis and so on. It is for the clinician to convert the problem in such a way that he is able to assess the likelihood of a disease process being present when certain symptoms appear. This is why the use of Bayes' theorem is so important when we look at medical decision making. It should help us to convert textbook knowledge into clinical situations. Seeing a patient who has a symptom such as a headache and knowing the incidence of headache in our patient population and in different disease processes, we should be able to predict the most likely diagnosis.

If we look at this outline in mathematical form we may state the problem more explicitly. If we denote the letter P as standing for probability of an event, we could say that $P(D)$ = probability of disease (D) being present in the population. We could write $P(D)$ = 0.01 if one person in every 100 of that population had disease D.

In the same way, $P(S)$ = probability of a symptom being present in a population of patients. Then, if we say $P(S|D)$ = probability of a symptom being present given that disease, we could write: $P(S|D)$ = 0.5 if half of all the patients with disease D had symptom S.

In a similar fashion, $P(D|S)$ = probability of a disease being present, given a particular symptom. Therefore, $P(D|S)$ = 0.25 would mean that a quarter of the patients with symptom S will have disease D.

We can take the converse of this by putting a bar over the notation, thus $\bar{D}$ or $\bar{S}$. This means that the disease is not present or the symptom is not present. Therefore, we could write: $P(\bar{S}|D)$ = 0.1 meaning that 10 per cent of people with disease D do not have symptom S. Finally, $P(\bar{D}|S)$ = 0.2 would mean that of those people who have symptom S, 20 per cent will not have disease D.

With all this in mind, we may now see how this information may be applied to an individual diagnosis. The patient presents with a symptom (S) and we wish to estimate the likelihood of a disease (D) being present, given that symptom: $P(D|S)$. For this calculation we need to know how often this particular symptom will be present in that particular disease: $P(S|D)$. This may be regarded as our understanding of the individual evidence. It is to be combined with the known incidence of the disease in the population: PD, and it will be divided by the known incidence of the symptom in the population:

PS. The resultant equation will appear as follows:

$$P(D|S) = (S|D) \cdot \frac{PD}{PS}.$$

If the disease is common, PD is large and therefore $P(D|S)$ will be high. It will be apparent that this is the equivalent of the old Oslerean aphorism that common things are common. If the symptom is common, PS will be large and therefore $P(D|S)$ will get smaller.

Closer scrutiny will tell us that for the equation to be useful, we need to add a little more to it. We shall need to know just how often the symptom S will be present in those members of the population who do not have disease, i.e. $\bar{D}$. This brings us back to our earlier discussion of the specificity and sensitivity of clinical features. We shall need to enlarge the equation to take all these considerations into account. We shall see that the significance of symptom S in the absence or presence of disease is affected by the frequency of D and of $\bar{D}$ in the population. If D is very rare and $\bar{D}$ is common and at the same time some patients have S in the absence of disease, then seeing a patient with symptom S will not have much effect on our initial probability estimate.

Our revised equation therefore may look like this:

$$P(D|S) = \frac{P(S|D) \cdot PD}{P(S|D) \cdot PD + P(S|\bar{D}) \cdot P\bar{D}}.$$

The new denominator in this slightly more complex equation takes into account not only the prevalence of D, but also $\bar{D}$, given a patient who has symptom S.

We may illustrate the working of this formula with the example of a disease D which may be a brain tumour. If we assume that this is seen in one in 1000 of the population then $PD = 0.001$.

This leaves $P\bar{D} = 0.999$.

If we say that 30 per cent of patients with a tumour have headaches (S) then $(S|D) = 0.3$.

Yet, we can also say that 20 per cent of the total population have headaches and, therefore, $PS = 0.2$.

Since most of these do not have a brain tumour, $P(S|\bar{D}) = 0.199$. The equation will therefore become:

$$P(D|S) = \frac{(0.3 \times 0.001)}{(0.3 \times 0.001) + (0.199 \times 0.999)} = 0.0015.$$

This means that the likelihood of the patient presenting with headache having a brain tumour is very low, hardly more than the disease prevalence in the population at large.

We can see how new evidence may alter this result. Let us say that our patient also has papilloedema, S_1. We may also make a few other assumptions:

$P(S_1|D) = 0.5$, which means that half those with brain tumours have papilloedema.

$P(S_1|\bar{D}) = 0.002$, so that one in 500 patients who have no brain tumour may have papilloedema.

$PD = 0.002$ we already know (we have rounded up from 0.0015 for ease of calculation). This is our new prior probability in patients who have headache i.e. $P(D|S)$ as calculated above.

$P\bar{D} = 0.998$ follows from this, i.e. probability of $\bar{D}$ if the patient has headache: $P(\bar{D}|S)$.

Therefore, the equation looks as follows:

$$P(D|S_1) = \frac{(0.5 \times 0.002)}{(0.5 \times 0.002) + (0.002 \times 0.998)} = 0.33.$$

This means that one-third of our patients with headache and papilloedema will have a brain tumour. Our initial probability estimate has now undergone a considerable revision to take into account the new information we obtained. To perform this calculation we assume that headache and papilloedema vary independently of each other. This implies that the presence of one does not affect the presence of the other. We shall return to this later.

Expected accuracy of predictions

This refers to the reliability of the individual data which will be used for altering our estimates. If we are going to revise our opinion and if we base this revision on some new data, we must assume that these are of good quality and reliability. Otherwise, we would be better off to stick to the basic rate of prior probability. Of course, if our knowledge of this is poor then predictions cannot be made.

The necessity for reliable data is a major criticism of the Bayesean approach to medical diagnosis. Probabilistic data are often unavailable and if they are, may be of poor reliability. This should not be a sufficient deterrent to our use of this model, but should allow us to make explicit the deficiencies in our knowledge. This approach helps us to recognize the information we require to make a reasonable guess at the diagnosis. If not available from our personal experience, it can frequently be found in the medical literature. Bayes' equation will also allow us to make calculations even in the absence of certain data, provided that we are able to demonstrate that the plausible values of such data will not materially affect our accuracy. At first sight this appears to be a difficult concept, but to illustrate it we return to our cerebral tumour suspect complaining of headaches.

Let us assume that we have no information about the frequency of headache in tumour patients. Under these circumstances we say $(S|D) = ?$

We have all the other information, so that the equation will be as follows:

$$P(D|S) = \frac{P(S|D) \cdot PD}{P(S|D) \cdot PD + P(S|\bar{D}) \cdot P\bar{D}}$$

$$= \frac{(? \times 0.001)}{(? \times 0.001) + (0.199 \times 0.999)}.$$

If we substitute values ranging from 0.1 to 0.9 for $P(S|D)$ we find that the value of $P(D|S)$ will vary from 0.001 to 0.004. In other words our results will hardly vary, no matter what we substitute for the question mark. The equation is insensitive $P(S|D)$ and so, even if we do not know the answer, it is irrelevant. We may therefore conclude that the Bayes equation helps us to sort out essential knowledge from that which is less important. Even if our knowledge base is imperfect, we can make reasonably accurate calculations.

Another problem, as we discussed in an earlier chapter, is that data obtained from patients could be unreliable. The patient's description of his sputum may be suggestive of haemoptysis but if we can actually see it for ourselves and analyse it in a laboratory, we would be on much safer grounds in using it as reliable information. The inexperienced observer may misinterpret the appearance of the optic fundus or of the plantar response. If he is aware of his deficiency he may seek more reliable information or even ignore his own findings until they are checked by someone else.

Correlations of data

We should also remember when revising opinions that new data may be correlated with previous information. Close correlation should not significantly affect changes brought about by the first set of information. For instance, consider a patient who complains of weight loss, has a goitre with a bruit over the gland, hot hands, a rapid bouncing pulse, proximal weakness and a tremor. There may also be heat intolerance, a good appetite and diarrhoea. All these features are very strongly correlated. Therefore, if we made a diagnosis of thyrotoxicosis on our original findings of weight loss, hyperactive circulation and thyroid bruit, the additional features mentioned should add little to our level of confidence.

Such correlations must always be taken into account when revising opinions about accuracy of predictions. We shall discuss this in more detail in the following section.

Possible diagnostic errors

When we use Bayesean analysis we need to watch for errors (Salamon *et al.* 1976), but the approach will also point out where clinicians are likely to make errors, irrespective of the diagnostic method they may be using (some of these will be discussed in more detail in Chapter 8).

Lack of accurate knowledge about prior probability or failure to take into account our knowledge of this prior probability. A group of neurologists and students was given a description of a patient with paraplegia and the various findings were slightly more consistent with a diagnosis of cord compression than with that of multiple sclerosis. At the same time, they were informed that the prior probability of the condition being multiple sclerosis was over 90 per cent. In spite of this, a large majority of subjects favoured a diagnosis of cord compression, completely ignoring the information about prior probability (Balla 1980*b*).

Lack of knowledge in perspective explains why students tend to pick on rare conditions when the experienced clinician will immediately diagnose something that tends to be more commonly seen by him.

Lack of change with new data. The main principle of the information processing approach is that early hypotheses should be formed. Some of these early hypotheses could be dependent on knowledge of prior probability.

We saw how errors may occur because of ignorance of this probability or because insufficient emphasis is placed on it. The opposite error of failing to change hypotheses with new information may apply equally. Several studies have shown that once a clinician has made up his mind about the diagnosis, he may ignore all contrary information and not take good evidence into account.

Accepting new data even though it may be of poor reliability. This is one of the major problems of the diagnostic process. In particular, the inexperienced will find it difficult to attach the correct weight to the information and to assess when it is reliable. For instance, a patient with slight backache who has symptoms of some muscular strain may be found to have an absent ankle jerk. As a result, the clinician may initiate multiple investigations, looking for a compressing lesion such as a lumbar disc protrusion. Careful reexamination by an expert may, however, show that the ankle jerks were present and that the technique of the original observer was at fault. As we said before, too much reliance on questionable technique may give an unwarranted increase in diagnostic confidence.

It is also apparent that emphasis is often placed on investigations with low specificity for the disease which is investigated. For instance, a patient who has non-specific abdominal pain may have a questionable area of calcification on a plain X-ray. This may be taken as strong evidence and further investigations may be carried out looking for a renal stone when the original clinical assessment would have suggested that the X-ray findings were likely to be of little significance. Undue reliance of some clinicians on special investigations is an important problem; not only specificity and sensitivity, but also observer error seem to be completely ignored when weighting the evidence.

The problem exemplified here has been referred to as 'the Ulysses Syndrome' (Rang 1972). As a result of unnecessary and uncritical investigations further tests are required to reassure doctor and patient of the irrelevance of the first, perhaps unexpected, abnormal result. This takes the patient on a long and at times hazardous journey of discovering that there is nothing wrong with him.

Ignoring the correlations between the various pieces of new data. When gathering new information, many clinicians tend to become more confident even though the extra information is worthless. For instance, a group of students was given a description of a patient with an extensor plantar response and of another patient with all the other associated clinical features of an upper motor neurone lesion. They felt that their confidence in the diagnosis of an upper motor neurone lesion was very much increased when the other features were also present. A group of neurologists tested with the same questions only showed a slight increase in confidence, being able to see the specificity of the extensor plantar response and lack of need for any other confirmation (Balla 1980*b*).

A study of expert gastroenterologists showed similar trends. Some experts gained increasing confidence from new data, even if they regarded these as being of little significance when asked to weight the cues independently. Simply having the information there, even if they regarded it as being relatively useless, gave them extra confidence (Balla *et al.* 1983).

Problems in relation to data correlation are especially important when we look at test ordering. This will be discussed in more detail in the Appendix (p. 135).

Two problem areas: utility and rarity

Even if we overcome all these problems, and a correct understanding of the Bayesian approach should help, there will still remain two areas which must cause concern. These relate to the concepts of utility and the need to retain the ability to diagnose rare events. In the clinical situation, our main concern is to increase utility and decrease risk to the individual patient, no matter how rare his disease may be. At times we may have to make a search for a rare, randomly occurring event which could be a high utility diagnosis. Finding a patient with Wilson's disease may be once in a lifetime even for the specialist, but the correct diagnosis would help to convert a physical cripple to normality. Bayes' theorem places a great deal of emphasis on prevalence and therefore, on purely probabilistic grounds, such a rarity may be missed. This could be acceptable to the health economist, but not to the clinician. The only possible way of diagnosing such rare events is by constant watchfulness. It is probable that some highly significant cue would alert us to the possible diagnosis. Then, we need to ignore all probabilistic calculations and concentrate on individual utility.

Unfortunately, this attitude is seen as being too extreme. Bayes' theorem should help to retain perspective in these cases. This means that the critical cue which alerted us to the diagnosis would need to be checked with extreme caution before proceeding with full investigations. For instance, the appearance of the brownish ring around the cornea may make us suspect Wilson's disease. Before arranging for complex biochemical tests, the exact nature of the discoloration should be looked at as a simple first procedure. It is probable that the attitude of careless acceptance of poor-quality data, combined with the constant and unreasonable search for rarities could explain a great deal of the excesses seen in investigative medicine.

The problem of utility of diagnosis may be solved by combining the measures of utility with the weight of the evidence. If, on purely probabilistic grounds, one diagnosis is suggested, and this diagnosis has little utility, others may also be entertained. We know that by far the commonest cause of chest pain would be musculo-skeletal in origin. We also know that cardiac pain may be of higher utility, if diagnosed at the appropriate time. Therefore, we include this less likely alternative in our data search. Once more, Bayes' theorem may guide and give perspective. It need not dictate our actions without further thought.

Gambles

It may be upsetting to consider the use of gambles when dealing with human life and of comparing medical decision making with a game of roulette or cards. Yet, an understanding of gambles, which link the taking of risks with the chance of winning, should be helpful in some decision-making situations (Payne 1973). When making a gamble four factors need to be considered and evaluated correctly. These are:

1 the probability of winning
2 the amount of likely win
3 the probability of losing
4 the amount of likely loss

These four risk factors need to be correctly identified and integrated, so that the right decisions may be made about the gamble. We would obviously like to win as much as possible and lose as little as possible. In medical decision making, losses tend to be of particular importance because we cannot 'afford' to make too many errors where a significant loss to the patient would be the result. For instance, if a patient presents with headache after a head injury, it is probable that these are simple post-concussional headaches which will settle over some weeks. There is also a possibility that he might be suffering from a subdural collection. If so, without treatment he will die. The diagnostic approach here revolves around the decision whether to investigate for a possible subdural collection. It is apparent that the probability of winning, in this case finding a subdural collection, is very small indeed. At the same time, the win would save his life. The probability of losing, of not finding an abnormality, is high, but a loss is death. Therefore, any significant chance of a loss must be eliminated because the loss would be too great. Investigations will therefore be carried out to exclude the unlikely possibility of a subdural collection.

A slight elaboration of this concept is that of '*duplex gambles*'. The basic idea behind this model is that if we have a choice of two approaches and if the probability of winning is greater than the probability of losing, we should pick the choice where the amount of the win is greater. In the alternative situation where the probability of winning is less, we should pick the choice with the smaller amount of loss. (Those familiar with the minimax principle may see certain similarities here.)

For instance, a patient with terminal cancer may develop paraplegia. Investigations and surgery would remove the immediate cause of the paraplegia, but death would not be delayed. There would also be increased discomfort in the post-operative phase. With the two alternatives of investigations and surgery or conservative management, most of us would tend to choose the one with the lesser loss, avoiding surgery and its possible post-operative discomfort.

Weighting of cues

Correct weighting of cues is the most fundamental part of decision making, without which it is impossible to make rational decisions (Coles *et al.* 1980). The weight attached to a cue refers to the subjective assessment of the significance of the data obtained by the doctor. It is assumed that this should, in turn, affect what sort of decisions will be made in the presence or absence of such cues. It must be apparent that some cues will be perceived as more significant than others, and we could then say that they were more heavily weighted than other data. This is what we mean by the scaling of cues. Accordingly, a strong or critical cue would be one which would strongly favour or negate one particular diagnostic alternative. As we have noted, such scaling of weights is rarely found in standard textbooks which are more likely to concentrate on lists of information.

Work by de Dombal *et al.* (1971) on abdominal pain has shown that it is possible to give weights to data so that diagnostic accuracy can be increased as a result. Similarly, Derouesné and colleagues in Paris (Salamon *et al.* 1976) have been collecting information on the significance of data for neurological diagnosis both in a retrospective and a prospective study. The findings indicate that individual judgments on the significance of clinical features will vary between clinicians and tend to be different from the results of prospective studies. It underlines the unreliability of so-called clinical impressions. A clinician may, for instance, think that he diagnoses coronary insufficiency on the quality of the pain, yet it could be shown that it is the timing of the symptom, rather than its quality or site, which is of more importance to him in coming to a diagnosis. It is clear that before it will be possible to make rational decisions in many clinical situations, a great deal more data must be collected so that proper weights can be assigned to different pieces of information.

To look at these ideas in more detail, a case vignette study was carried out, using cardiologists, neurologists and students as subjects (Balla 1982). Brief case histories were given with a variable number of cues in each case. One case concerned a patient with olfactory sensations and *déjà vu*, both of which are strong cues for epilepsy. All other indicators for epilepsy were specifically noted as being absent. It was found that most subjects diagnosed epilepsy and that preference for this diagnosis increased with expertise. These findings would suggest that with increasing expertise in the field, subjects are more likely to perceive the most heavily weighted cues. Another case described a patient with convulsions, tongue biting and incontinence, the commonly accepted classic features of epileptic seizures. Additional cues included that he had been drinking and felt ill before collapsing. Neurologists generally did not diagnose this as an epileptic fit, but other groups did. This indicated that different speciality groups attached differing weights to cues. Thus, neurologists must have regarded the preceding circumstances and symptoms more important than any other cues, in contrast to the other specialists and students. This raises one important issue about the weighting of cues. One possibility is that specialists know more about the intrinsic nature of a problem than others. The alternative explanation is that different groups of doctors will give differing definitions of the same situation. This brings us back to the problem of the unfalsifiable diagnosis, where the definition given by the doctor determines the nature of the case. This can certainly explain why so many patients will have multiple diagnostic labels where they present the same problem to different doctors.

There would be little doubt that negative information is generally difficult to handle, yet it will contain critical cues. It will frequently be ignored by the inexperienced, though experts may place a lot of importance on it. For instance, temporal arteritis and polymyalgia rheumatica are diseases of the elderly, whilst the onset of petit mal is confined to childhood. Therefore, headache in a young man would not be caused by arteritis, and a first blackout in a patient of 50 years could not be petit mal. Yet, a large number of clinicians ignore this evidence even when they are aware of the age-specific incidence of these conditions.

The next step will be *integration* of the various cues so that the weights can be assessed in individual situations. We must learn that the significance of the diagnostic cues will vary depending on the setting. One of the most important influences here will be the prior probability of disease being present with different frequencies depending on the general background of the patient. We may cite the example mentioned earlier of haemoptysis in a Western country being a strong cue for bronchitis, yet, in the Third World it may be a strong cue for tuberculosis.

In a study of episodic blackouts, case vignettes were drawn up in which three patients with typical fainting spells were described (Balla 1982). One was a young girl who blacked out in church, and another was a person from a much older age group. The third case had no information on age or sex of the patient. In the case of the girl there was a high score for vaso-vagal episodes because of the knowledge that these were common in this age group. For the patient in the older age group, where such episodes would be somewhat less common, a much less confident diagnosis was given. In the third case where no prior information was given, many of the subjects were unable to make an accurate guess. This shows that the same information in three different settings would have completely different weights, and that this would be influenced by prior information.

The work of Anderson (1972) on what he called configurality in clinical judgment is also consistent with these findings. Anderson felt that the most important method used by clinicians when assessing pieces of information was to average the weights before expressing judgment. It has also been shown that when data are correlated many clinicians have difficulty in assessing how this correlation will affect the final decisions. The example quoted earlier, of correlation between the different clinical features of an upper motor neurone lesion, illustrates this. In spite of the strong correlation, many subjects tend to show increasing confidence in their decisions as they obtain the data which will be highly correlated in the first place and where the final judgment should not, therefore, have been affected by the extra information available (Balla 1980*b*). It is generally not understood that such additional data may only correlate with the previously obtained clinical features and does not enhance specificity for the disease itself.

The need to learn the correct weights of cues is self-evident. The cursory attempts made to teach these in textbooks are unacceptable. The recent trend towards quantifying medical knowledge will help in the long run. Until then, students will still need to understand the significance of scaling and integration of cues. Learning patterns of diseases may be helpful, but understanding how to weight cues and, in particular, learning to perceive incongruous evidence are essential.

We have made previous reference to specificity and sensitivity of clinical features as being useful for weighting our data. We can now go further and introduce the concept of the predictive value of information. We need to measure the weight of our data and show how it is combined with our understanding of the prevalence of the disease. In order to do this, we shall need to introduce and define a few more terms.

These concepts, though superficially simple, may be difficult for students to grasp. Some find it easier with the use of 2 × 2 tables. If we have disease (*D*) in the columns and clinical feature (*X*) in the rows, the table appears as shown in Table 7.1.

We see that there will be cases where the clinical feature and the disease coexist and we refer to these as true positive (*TP*). At the other end of the scale are cases where neither the disease nor the clinical feature exist and these are the true negatives (*TN*). When the disease is present, but the test is negative, we obtain a false negative (*FN*). When the disease is absent, but the test is positive, then the result is a false positive (*FP*). According to our notation in the 2 × 2 table, one column contains all the disease cases, and these consist of *TP* and *FN* adding up to the total cases of disease. The other column contains all the non-disease cases, consisting of *FP* and *TN*, adding up to the total cases of non-disease. In the first row we see all the cases of positive tests, comprising *TP* and *FP*. The second row is made up of all the negative tests, consisting of *FN* and *TN*.

Fig. 7.1 demonstrates this in a different form which can then be put in a 2 × 2 table (Table 7.2).

Table 7.1. *2 × 2 table to show true positive (TP), false positive (FP) true negative (TN), false negative (FN)*

	D^+	D^-	
X^+	TP	FP	Total positive test
X^-	FN	TN	Total negative test
	Total disease	Total no disease	Total tested

Fig. 7.1. Population of squares (*n* = 50), showing those with disease *D* (*n* = 5) and clinical feature *X* (*n* = 10).

	D								
		D							
X	X	X	X	X	D X	X	D X	X	X
									D

True positive (*TP*) indicates that the test is positive in the presence of disease. It is the probability of a patient with D also having X: $P(X|D)$. We note that this is related to *sensitivity* which may be expressed as follows:

$$\text{sensitivity} = \frac{\text{true positive}}{\text{total disease (i.e. } TP + FN)} \times 100.$$

This refers to the proportion of patients with disease who have the abnormality we are looking for.

If a test is highly sensitive (has a high true positive rate), then a negative test result is a good predictor of the absence of disease. Such tests may therefore be good for screening populations.

We may take the example of a patient who has facial pain strictly within the anatomical distribution of the trigeminal nerve. We know that this is the distribution of pain in all patients with trigeminal neuralgia, but in 10 per cent of other cases, for instance dental neuralgia, pain could be in a similar anatomical distribution. (We may put this in the form of symbolic notation a follows: $A|N = 1$, $A|O = 0.1$, where A is the anatomical distribution of the pain, N refers to trigeminal neuralgia and O to other types of pain.) In a 2×2 table format we derive Table 7.3. This tells us that if the patient has pain outside the trigeminal nerve distribution it cannot be trigeminal neuralgia because there are no false negatives in the table. In has clearly been a good predictor of the absence of disease.

Table 7.2. *2 × 2 table derived from Fig. 7.1*

	D	$\bar{D}$	
X	2	8	10
$\bar{X}$	3	37	40
Total	5	45	50

More have clinical feature (X) without disease ($\bar{D}$) than in the presence of disease (D).

Table 7.3. *Table demonstrating a test with sensitivity of 100 per cent*

	N	O
A^+	1.0	0.1
A^-	0	0.9

It will be apparent that to calculate sensitivity, we divide *TP* by the column total.

True negative (*TN*) indicates that the test should be negative in health. It is the probability of a patient with D^- not having X: $P(\bar{X}|\bar{D})$. This is a reflection of *specificity* which is shown in the following equation.

$$\text{specificity} = \frac{\text{true negative}}{\text{total non-disease (i.e. } TN + FP)} \times 100.$$

This proportion of patients with the negative test is non-diseased. If the test is highly specific, then it would indicate that few without the disease would have an abnormal test. For instance, if we are given information that crushing chest pain is present in 80 per cent of patients with coronary artery disease, but in only five per cent of those with other causes of chest pain, we can put it in a format as in Table 7.4 (in symbolic notations: $C|MI = 0.8$, $C|O = 0.05$, where *C* refers to crushing chest pain, *MI* to coronary disease, *O* to other causes of the pain). To obtain specificity, we divided *TN* by the column total.

Predictive values of tests

From here we may go on to to combine our knowledge of the prior probability of the disease with the above estimates and we shall see how the weight of our information will change significantly depending on its setting.

It must be made clear that all the above terms refer to patients

Table 7.4. *Table demonstrating a test with a specificity of 95 per cent*

	MI	O
C^+	0.8	0.05
C^-	0.2	0.95

who have the disease. *Sensitivity* (or true positive rate) is the probability that the test will be positive when given to a person with the disease. This means that if the true positive rate is 90 per cent, then 90 per cent of diseased patients will have that clinical feature. It does not take into account those members of the population who do not have the disease. *Specificity* (or true negative rate) will mean that the test will be negative when given to patient who does not have the disease. Therefore, once more the significance of this true negative rate is affected by the proportion of patients who have the disease in the population we are looking at.

In any population, some individuals suffer from the disease under consideration, and some do not. Therefore, we must use another set of calculations to assess the significance of the test result (or clinical feature) in predicting the presence or absence of disease. This is where a knowledge of the prevalence of disease in the population becomes important. Many will find it difficult to comprehend how the same test result may have a completely different significance in different populations. We shall give an example using a 2 × 2 table. If we take a disease (D) with 90 per cent true negatives (specificity) and also 90 per cent true positives (sensitivity), and a prevalence rate of one in 100 in a hypothetical sample of 1000 patients, the table will be as shown in Table 7.5.

Looking at the table we may see how the various results were obtained. There are 10 patients with D, and since the test is positive in 90 per cent of them, there will be nine *TP* and one *FN*. This leaves us with 990 patients without disease ($\bar{D}$), but since the test is only

Table 7.5. *A sample of 1000 hypothetical patients with one per cent disease prevalence*

	D	$\bar{D}$	Total
C	9	99	108 (Total positive test)
	(*TP*)	(*FP*)	
$\bar{C}$	1	891	892 (Total negative test)
	(*FN*)	(*TN*)	
	10	990	1000
	(Total disease)	(Total no disease)	(Total tested)

90 per cent specific, there will be 10 per cent of these 990 who will have a positive result in the absence of disease. This will give us 99 *FP*.

A glance through the table will show that there are more false positives than true positives and so we come to an understanding of what we mean by a predictive value of a test. To obtain this value, we must know not only how many true positives there will be, but also how many false positives we obtained:

$$\text{predictive value positive} = \frac{\text{true positive}}{\text{total positive}}$$

$$= \frac{9}{108} = 0.08.$$

In other words, we understand that if one of our patients in this hypothetical sample has a positive result for clinical feature *C*, he will have an eight per cent chance of having the disease, and 92 per cent will be false positives. A *positive predictive value* is therefore the probability that a person with a positive test result will have the disease.

We note that the predictive value positive was calculated by dividing the *TP* by the row total.

The value of a negative test result can be calculated in a similar way:

$$\text{predictive value negative} = \frac{\text{true negative}}{\text{total negative}}$$

$$= \frac{891}{892} = 0.998.$$

This shows us that a negative test result in this case will in fact have a high predictive value. A *negative predictive value* may therefore be seen as the probability that a person with a negative test result will not have the disease. In this example, it again underlines the great importance that may at times be attached to negative information, in contrast to the relatively small value of the positive information that was obtained.

To illustrate further how, in an example containing the same specificity and sensitivity of clinical information, a change in prevalence will alter the weight of the information we obtain, we may take the same hypothetical 1000 patients, but this time assume a disease prevalence rate of 20 per cent. Table 7.6 shows the results we will now obtain.

$$\text{Predictive value positive} = \frac{180}{260} = 0.69.$$

$$\text{Predictive value negative} = \frac{720}{740} = 0.97.$$

We see that now the predictive value for positive clinical features is close to 70 per cent.

In view of the significant shifts in predictive value according to the population studies, and unless we know the prevalence of the disease in our population, we must always interpret tests with caution. It is useful to select sub-populations for study if we wish to

Table 7.6. *A sample of 1000 hypothetical patients with 20 per cent disease prevalence*

	D	D̄	Total
C	180	80	260
C̄	20	720	740
	200	800	1000

avoid the problems created by large numbers of false positive tests. An example of this will be given in the Appendix (p. 137).

These are indeed very difficult concepts for most students and doctors to assimilate and, as we mentioned earlier, textbook knowledge does not really help here. There are wide gaps in knowledge and in particular understanding of false positive and true negative rates is lacking (J. Balla and M. Holmes, unpublished observations). Studies both of expert clinicians (Berwick *et al.* 1981) and of medical students (Balla, Elstein & Gates 1983) have shown a general lack of understanding of all these terms resulting in haphazard use of the information which is presented to them.

Decision trees

The last topic to be pursued will concern decision trees. These are the 'fundamental analytical tool of decision analysis' (Weinstein & Fineberg 1980). They may appear unduly burdensome and at first sight frightening in their complexity. However, they may be used to display a logical temporal sequence of decision making. Their availability should allow for revision of entrenched 'opinion'. They may also be used for exploring the apparently illogical. Therefore, students should be conversant with some of the fundamental principles governing their use. Only the most rudimentary outline will be given here and readers who wish to go further should consult a more advanced book on decision analysis such as Weinstein & Fineberg (1980).

When we are faced with making choices amongst alternatives *A* and *B* we may visualize our possible courses of action as being along the branches of a tree:

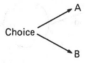

We may then see that there are two ways that these alternatives may eventuate. The first of these concerns the possibility that we have some say in the matter, and that we make a conscious decision about which alternative we would prefer. By convention, we call this a '*decision node*' and symbolize it with a square box on the tree:

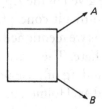

If we have no say as to which alternative will appear, then it becomes a '*chance node*', and it is denoted by a circle:

An example of the former may be to perform a CT scan on the brain, and of the latter would be the finding of a brain tumour, whether the tests were performed or not. This would clearly be beyond our control, and therefore a matter of chance.

Thus, if we wish to have a tree for brain tumours being tested with a CT scan, the decision tree may appear as follows:

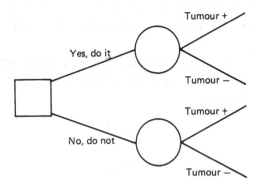

The way this tree becomes useful is by attaching probabilities to each branch. Then we should be able to select the course which will lead us to the most valued outcome, in this case, the finding of a brain tumour.

If we now enlarge the tree, and assume that there is a clinical feature (*W*) which is also present, and it may affect the probability of a tumour (*T*) being found, four new branches will appear:

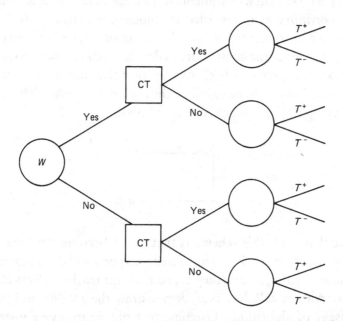

If we attach the new probabilities to each branch, we should see which combination is going to lead to finding the most tumours and missing the least. At the same time, it will also tell us how many negative tests we should perform. If our aim is to find the most tumours with the least number of tests, our course of action will be clearly and logically mapped out by this method.

Now, we did not put any figures into the above examples because the calculation of the various probability estimates can be a complex task. For the interested reader we attach one example in the Appendix (p. 139) and other excellent illustrations are available in *Clinical Decision Analysis* (Weinstein & Fineberg 1980).

If the task is somewhat complex, it may not be a suitable method for everyday clinical use. There are those who believe that because of the advantages of computer technology, mathematical complexity need not be a deterrent. It is difficult to accept this, and it is suggested here that complex trees may well be replaced by *algorithms*. There is evidence to suggest that expert clinicians do use such combinations of rules of thumb. They learn this by experience, but there is no reason why students should not be able to use them.

An *algorithm* may be regarded as a much pruned tree, with all the unattractive branches lopped off. It is a set of rules which may be followed to reduce the complexity of decision making. For instance, in the example given earlier, we may find that the most suitable course of action would be to follow the topmost branches. Then, we may develop a simple set of rules as follows:

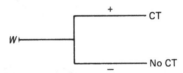

The problem with this scheme is that it can become a vehicle for thoughtless, repetitive behaviour. Many experts will deny that they ever use such rules, or that they are suitable for teaching. Reflection and observation will, however, demonstrate the validity and common usage of algorithms. Listening to a physician giving instructions in the management of diabetes is one example: 'If the blood glucose is over 300 mg in four hours, then give another dose of insulin. If it is below this, then wait another four hours. Then, if there is glycosuria, repeat the blood sugar' . . . and so on. Surely this is a classic use of an algorithm. He must have developed it through experience, and is now passing it on to patients, nurses and students.

Such algorithms may be developed retrospectively, and the results of certain accepted forms of management may be questioned and compared with results obtained using criteria that have been developed from a decision analytic approach. For instance, an algorithm was obtained for the management of urinary incontinence and it was shown that it would lead to 60 per cent reduction of invasive investigations (Hilton & Stanton 1981). Another study of the use of skull X-rays and CT scans in head-injured patients (detailed in the Appendix) also demonstrated that there is a need to question present forms of management and that the use of investigations may be put on a rational basis (Balla & Elstein 1984). The multiplicity of tests used for the diagnosis of pancreatic disease can also be put in the form of an algorithm by this method, thus reducing the cost and complexity of investigations (Braganza 1982).

The use of formal decision trees is advocated here to explain to students how the various rules were developed, and to scrutinize decision making as new knowledge, techniques and treatments develop. This kind of periodic review would then prevent medicine from becoming a static technology and allow persistent questioning and constant attempts at falsification.

It is also apparent that these decision analytic techniques allow us to look at the ethical issues in decision making. We can now make explicit the nature of the risk taken when pursuing certain forms of action (Brett 1981). Decision analysis is no panacea for all our problems, but it helps to highlight them and aids us in a better understanding of our activities.

Summary

Many of the points raised in this section are summarized in Fig. 7.2. The degree of certainty of the diagnosis is shown on the vertical axis and the amount of data obtained is shown on the horizontal. Prior probability, shown as point *A* on the horizontal, will usually be the

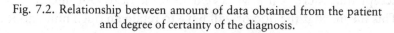

Fig. 7.2. Relationship between amount of data obtained from the patient and degree of certainty of the diagnosis.

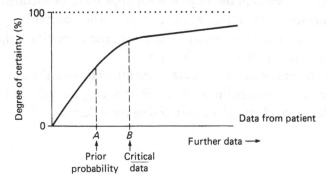

most heavily weighted information. Thus, knowledge of prior probability will in many instances lead to a reasonably accurate guess at the diagnosis. New specific evidence about the individual case should then increase the degree of confidence in this diagnosis. From point *A* to point *B* on the horizontal are shown the important new data which may be obtained. This refers to the most heavily weighted evidence. As seen on the vertical axis, in most instances this will not give absolute certainty about the diagnosis. A decision will then have to be made on whether further data need to be obtained beyond *B*. These data will usually be more expensive to obtain, and calculations of the relevant risk of not having a certain diagnosis, versus the utility of closer approximation to certainty, will help us to decide whether it is necessary to look for further cues. It is evident that in most cases it will be important for students to learn about prior probability and also about the heavily weighted cues. They will also need to understand when to stop collecting data.

If we are to review some of these points within the perspective of the proper scientific orientation, the need for careful evaluation of data immediately becomes evident. The data used for hypothesis testing must be reliable, and the best information will be that which can be used in attempts at falsification. Thus, negative information will often be most heavily weighted and should be sought in preference to the accumulation of positive data. As a corollary, all diagnostic hypotheses must be testable, and the clinician will have to accept that there will always remain some degree of uncertainty. This means that the doctor will have to retain an open mind about the diagnosis, even in the face of what appears to be incontrovertible evidence in favour of his hypothesis. The constant need for utility consideration is also apparent from the admonition that we should not seek precision for its own sake.

Readers who wish to become more familiar with the use of the mathematical concepts introduced in this chapter will find three examples in the Appendix at the end of the volume.

8
Decision making
DESCRIPTIVE MODELS
℣

We saw in the previous section how an idealised diagnostician would behave if he had a perfect understanding of how to handle evidence and how to make decisions. In that chapter, we indicated that such rules were rarely followed by real-life clinicians, though an understanding of these rules may help to improve performance and reduce sources of error. In the following pages, it will be our aim to see how decisions are made in everyday situations and how these may be related to the work of the clinician. We shall describe models of decision rules used in real-life decision making and stress some of the systematic errors which occur due to the various inbuilt biases of decision makers. An understanding of the rules helps us as teachers to observe and analyse the reasons behind our clinical decisions. This should be valuable in explaining our actions to students. In particular, the modelling of the choices in our minds is useful in leading us to an understanding of what is important information for students to learn and to observe.

Most descriptive studies on decision making come from outside the field of medicine and there has been little empirical work to show how diagnostic decisions are made in clinical practice. With a great deal of insight Dudley (1968) was one of the first to suggest that we may be using different rules depending on the task in hand. He referred to those of heuristics, pattern recognition and pay-offs. We shall see that these predictions were close to the truth, though even today we are just beginning to have a glimmer of understanding of how the clinician's mind works. It is not suggested that clinicians consciously think according to these rules. These are merely models which explain decision making and give insights into the process.

When dealing with descriptive models, we shall first have to see how the available choices are represented in the subject's mind. Then, we shall see what sort of decision rules are available to make these choices and how the rules may be combined in particular situations (Montgomery & Svenson 1976). We attempt to see the reasons behind making decisions and, finally, what sort of rules of thumb may be available to ease the burden of decision making. Though most studies come from fields outside medicine (Svenson 1974) a look at these models may give us some ideas on how the clinician may be performing, and generalizations from one field to another will have to be made. We shall deal with descriptive theory under the following headings:

1 The subjective representation of choice
2 The decision rules that are available
3 How these rules are chosen and combined
4 Systematic errors

Subjective representation of choice

If we are asked to make a choice among a number of *alternatives*, each of the alternatives can be described as having a number of different aspects (Montgomery & Svenson 1976). (Unfortunately, terms are not always clearly defined and in much of the literature the words 'aspect' and 'attribute' may at times be interchanged.) We see that some of the *aspects* may be compared with each other. An aspect may appear more attractive on one alternative than on the other, so that we should be able to measure attractiveness on a scale and attach values to it. We can therefore say that an aspect will have a certain value which is a measure of *attractiveness*. We may take the example of choosing a car. Cost may be one aspect and value here would be easy to measure on an interval scale of attractiveness. Another aspect of a car would be its petrol consumption and again this would be an easy measure in kilometres per litre which could in its own turn be expressed in monetary terms. A third aspect of the same car may be its colour and now we can see that measurement of values is more difficult, but we know that one individual may find yellow more attractive than red so that for this particular person a yellow car would have a higher value of attractiveness on the aspect of colour than a red car.

We can translate this to a situation where alternative choices may be that a patient is suffering from multiple sclerosis or from a spinal cord tumour. If this patient is paraplegic, then this is one aspect of his condition. We know that both multiple sclerosis and a spinal cord tumour may cause weak legs; therefore, the value (attractiveness) of paraplegia would be about equal for both diagnostic choices. If the same patient has a fluctuating course, then we know that this aspect would be in favour of a diagnosis of multiple sclerosis, whereas a progressive steady decline would be a more attractive choice for diagnosing a spinal cord tumour. If we can understand that the term 'value' under these conditions is no more than a measure of attractiveness for a particular choice, then we should be able to apply such measures when studying the diagnostic process.

Decision rules

These vary from relatively low to relatively high complexity (Montgomery & Sevnson 1976). We shall do no more than outline the principles behind a few of these rules, at the same time emphasizing once more that there is almost no published work on medical decision making to show whether these rules are applicable to the diagnostic process.

Ordinal measures of attractiveness

An ordinal scale refers to categories which cannot be put into a very clear numerical sequence. For instance, one could say that a house is bigger or is further away from the railway station than an alternative choice. No actual measurements are given, it is just a relatively rough hierarchical scaling. We can see that these rules could be used when attractiveness is measured on an ordinal scale. The simplest of these rules is the so-called *dominance rule* which states that if alternative *A* is better than alternative *B* *on at least one aspect and not worse than the other alternative on any other aspect, then alternative A* will be chosen. If we find that house *A* is closer to the station than house *B* and that both houses are the same size, with the same number of bedrooms, and we are not interested in any other aspects, then we shall choose house *A*. With ordinal rules of this kind, it is often difficult to make a clear choice because of lack of sufficient information of significant distinguishing values between the two choices.

We could think of an example where this rule may be favoured, for instance, when looking at a cavity on a chest X-ray. The choice may be between tuberculosis or carcinoma and the size and shape of the cavity would be acceptable for both diagnostic possibilities. If the cavity is in the upper lobe, it can be regarded as an aspect in favour of tuberculosis and this would be a provisional diagnostic choice with the understanding that a great deal more information will be required to make a definite decision.

The *conjunctive rule* is a slightly more complicated version of ordinal measurements where it is stated that attractiveness of every aspect on the chosen alternative must exceed some sort of criterion whilst the alternative that will not be chosen should fall below this criterion on at least one aspect. The house that is chosen should exceed a certain number of rooms, distance from the station and price, whereas the one that is not chosen is the same price and distance, but falls below the requirements on size.

The prerequisite for using this rule is that the alternatives can be compared on the chosen aspects. If both alternatives have aspects with values above the chosen criteria, the choice will not be possible.

Rank-ordering of attractiveness

This rule requires that aspects are rank-ordered in terms of importance. Then, the choice alternative will be the one with the most attractive value on the most important aspect. For instance, when buying a house, a prospective purchaser may decide that the most important measure is the number of bedrooms and that nothing else matters. Then, when making a choice, he looks at the number of bedrooms; if this falls below the required number, there is no point in looking further and other aspects will not even be examined.

A variation on this theme is the *elimination by aspect* rule of Tversky (1972). This rule differs from the others in that comparisons do not have to be made in any special sort of order, but at every stage aspects are selected for comparison and choices made for the alternative which does not include the selected aspect. Thus, aspects which are common to all the alternatives under consideration will not affect the choice. Elimination continues until a single attractive aspect is found which is present on one choice alternative, but not on the others. This is a particularly useful rule because not just the overall value of a single aspect is considered, but also what is more important, its relationships to other aspects in the alternative choices. It is, therefore, easier to make a clear-cut choice without having to rely on an estimate of relative weights which so many people find difficult. It can be regarded as a useful simplification procedure, the major drawback being the assumption that the aspect which was picked as having distinguishing value was correct and relevant, and superior to the ones that were eliminated.

We can use this rule both in a sense of excluding possibilities or of including them as our favourite choice. For instance, given the knowledge that polymyalgia rheumatica is a disease affecting older age groups, we would not entertain the diagnosis in a child. The value of the age aspect of our patient would immediately exclude this diagnostic alternative.

The major pitfall of this way of decision making will be the problem faced in making a correct choice of the aspect whose value will be regarded as being of greatest importance. For instance, on seeing a patient with post-traumatic headache, the alternatives considered were that he was either having post-concussional headaches or that these were related to a subdural collection. Knowing that subdural blood clots tend to induce a changing and fluctuating conscious state, the clinician regarded this as the most important distinguishing criterion. Accordingly, a diagnosis of post-concussional headache was made and further investigations were not ordered. On listening to the story a little more closely, it became apparent that the patient complained of increasingly severe headache and from this point of view the condition appeared to be getting worse. Had this particular aspect been taken into consideration, the correct diagnosis of a subdural blood clot would have been made in the first instance. This case illustrates how we need to make continuous reassessment of what are the important aspects for making particular choices so that grave diagnostic errors may be avoided when using this kind of decision rule. Similar problems have been reported concerning the diagnosis of myocardial infarction (Leader, *The Lancet* 1982). In doubtful cases there remains considerable disagreement amongst experts about the weighting of aspects. As a result, in 100 such cases three experts could only agree on 42 diagnoses using their 'clinical instincts'.

Interval scale rules

This is a matter of adding up the values of the different pieces of information and then choosing the alternative with the highest total value. It is likely that this type of simple rule is used in a number of situations, but again, there is little empirical evidence to prove it. Even more simplified forms of this type of decision rule may be used when making decisions on certain forms of treatment. For instance, before deciding on the need for angiography and surgery in cases of cerebral vascular disease, we gave different values to various aspects such as age, the presence or absence of a carotid bruit as well as blood pressure (Balla unpublished observations). The values were added up and those patients who reached a certain figure were subjected to angiography whilst those who fell below it were given anticoagulants. We found that we were able to make relatively consistent treatment decisions following this protocol.

The choice of decision rules

To test these models in a clinical setting, we carried out two studies using simulated patients. In the first of these (Balla 1981), five expert neurologists and twelve students were given a case of multiple sclerosis. This could be regarded as a relatively easy diagnostic problem where the major distinction was to be made between multiple sclerosis and a spinal cord tumour. In both these conditions paraplegia and sphincter disturbance are aspects which would not have great distinguishing value as they could occur with either disease. We then looked at the course of the disease and regarded this as another aspect, a fluctuating course being present with multiple sclerosis, but not with the other choice alternative. We found that the clinicians examined relatively few aspects and after they evaluated what they regarded as significant data they made few changes to their diagnostic hypothesis. This type of behaviour on the part of the decision maker would be consistent with the use of the dominance rule. According to this, the aspect 'episodic nature' was the only one valued in favour of the diagnosis of multiple sclerosis, which was made by most of the clinicians.

Another rule which could explain the decision equally well is Tversky's elimination by aspect rule. In this instance the aspect which determines the choice is the one which will only be seen in a single alternative, but not in the others. Assuming again that 'episodic nature' is the significant aspect, we may understand why the subjects tended to ignore the remaining available information which did not seem to support the diagnosis of multiple sclerosis. We may speculate that the one expert and the three students who came to the wrong diagnosis were unable to assess the importance of this aspect and did not attach sufficient weight to it.

In our next study (Balla 1983) we looked at the difficult diagnostic problem of a patient with blackouts (Fig. 8.1). This was an interesting problem to explore in that it helped us to understand what makes a diagnostic problem difficult. The two major alternative diagnoses considered here were epilepsy or cardiac syncope. Loss of consciousness could be one aspect, clearly present in both alternatives. Palpitations may be another aspect tending to favour

Fig. 8.1. Decision rules.

Dominance rule:

If $A > B$ on 1(+) aspect,
choose A.
e.g. Erect posture, choose faint.

Conjunctive rule:

If $A > x$ on all aspects,
and $B < x$ on 1(+) aspect,
choose A.
e.g. No cardiac symptoms, not cardiac

Elimination by aspect:

If, $Ax + B\bar{x} \rightarrow A$
and $A\bar{x} \rightarrow \bar{A}$
e.g. Asystole, choose cardiac,
but no asystole does not exclude.

cardiac disease. Each of these aspects would then have a number of values so that palpitation may be regular, irregular or slow. Fourteen experts were examined and it was apparent that they used various decision rules. Most of them seemed to use the dominance rule. They stated that the classic epileptic features were more attractive for epilepsy than for other alternatives. A number of subjects used the conjunctive rule as implied by their statement that since cardiac markers were absent, they preferred epilepsy or faint as their choice. Most had very low levels of diagnostic confidence which is to be expected in the use of dominance or conjunctive rules where the fine differentiation of cue weights has to be relied on, as opposed to using a single critical distinguishing cue to make the alternative choice. It may therefore be concluded that the cues available in this type of case do not lend themselves to the use of some otherwise satisfactory decision rules such as the elimination by aspect rule of Tversky.

This study highlighted the need for finding heavily weighted distinguishing criteria to make an accurate and confident diagnosis. In conditions where such criteria are absent, diagnostic confidence will remain low and diagnosis unreliable. This problem was further stressed in another study on the diagnostic process of gastroenterologists (Balla *et al.* 1983). We found that the experts tended to attach different weights to a number of cues and, in particular, each expert tended to deviate from the norm on at least one cue weight assessment. Since the accurate assessment of data weights is important if decision rules are to be used with any degree of confidence, this may be an explanation for variation in diagnoses reached or the method of diagnosis used by experts even within the same field.

This view of decision making demonstrates the significant differences which exist between the idealized mathematical, as opposed to descriptive, models. We need to ask why individuals use these simplified rules. Is it simply a matter of being easy to use, or is it that the more complex rules, even if they give greater accuracy, are deemed unnecessary? If this were the case, it would indicate that any loss of accuracy was a reasonable trade-off in terms of time saved and the general accuracy of using a simple cognitive device (Thorngate 1980). If so, this would be consistent with the suggestion of Popper (1972) that increased precision for its own sake is of no benefit in any scientific endeavour.

In the context of medical diagnosis, we shall have to consider whether, as a result of changing attitudes and knowledge, rules which were satisfactory at one stage of the evolution of medicine might become outmoded at another point in time. Non-falsifiable diagnosis and non-specific therapy may be acceptable at one time, but not at another. In the days when tuberculosis and carcinoma of the lung were untreatable, a vague diagnosis of chest disease may have been satisfactory. When at least one of these conditions becomes eminently treatable, it may be necessary to reconsider decision-making strategies. Similar considerations apply to the introduction of new technologies. For instance, CT scanning has revolutionized the management of head injuries. Whereas previously clinicians would have had to rely on the interpretation of clinical signs and of skull X-rays, these criteria may in many instances be of relatively little value as opposed to changes on CT scans. In order to use decision rules with any degree of validity we need techniques to evaluate these new methods and this may at times require formal decision analytic methods. In a study we carried out on the indications for CT scans and skull X-rays in head-injured patients (Balla & Elstein 1984) we were able to develop a new algorithm (Fig. 8.2). The clinician needs to know what value to

Fig. 8.2. Head injury algorithm.

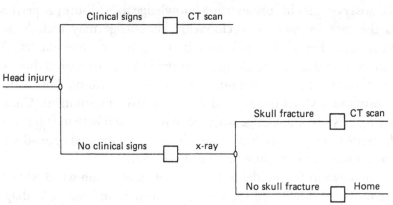

attach to the various aspects under consideration and accordingly should then change the decision rules that he had been using in the past. Such regular review of decision making is essential in an age of fast-changing technology and new therapeutic developments as well as the appearance of hitherto unknown diseases. This brings us to the next problem in the study of decision making, which is the integration of the available decision rules.

Integration procedures

It is evident that different rules may be used according to the task in hand and also according to the individual characteristics of the decision maker. The choice of decision rules and information-processing techniques, therefore, will be extremely variable, but we should still be able to see some sort of guiding principle behind individual decision making. The concept of *cognitive control*, as introduced by Hammond and Summers (1972), helps our understanding of the subject. It is assumed that the decision maker will be able to attach correct weights to his decisions and will be able to see the utility of his choices. Cognitive control assumes that the decision maker is able to use his knowledge consistently and 'usefully'. Earlier on, we discussed the importance of encyclopaedic knowledge and especially the correct structuring of this knowledge so that it is in a useful form. It is a matter then of integrating this usable knowledge with the information obtained from the task environment, so that useful decisions can be made.

Such decisions will clearly be based on inference, a method where the observer uses his pre-existing knowledge to attribute properties to the task in hand. Encyclopaedic knowledge may include an awareness that abdominal pain is a feature of appendicitis. A patient may them come along and provide the information that he has abdominal pain and a number of other symptoms. This is the information which is obtained from the task environment. Combining existing knowledge with the new data will help us infer that the patient does indeed have appendicitis. The inflamed appendix is not actually seen: its presence is only inferred.

We may put this model in the form of an equation which shows the interaction between the subject (clinician) and the task (diagnosis), demonstrating the relative importance of knowledge and of technique in coming to an accurate decision. Technique in this model represents the subject's internal activities in drawing certain inferences from the data. A version modified after Hammond & Summers (1972) would look like this:

$$A = K E T$$

A: We could term this diagnostic accuracy or a measure of correct decision making.

K: This is a measure of the subject's knowledge of the task. Specifically, it refers to the useful knowledge that is available and that can be used for decision making. If a clinician sees a patient with thyroid disease, he will need to know that there may be weight loss, heat intolerance, rapid circulation and an enlarged thyroid gland. It is this important, heavily weighted information that we must concentrate on teaching to students.

E: This refers to the inherent difficulty of the particular task. Some situations will be more predictable than others. We know for instance, that in some areas where weather patterns are stable, forecasting will be easy, but in others where there is great variability, the task will be inherently more difficult and errors will be at a much higher rate than in the stable situation. Similarly, some diseases will be more easily diagnosed than others, so that flexural eczema will be easily picked, simply by looking at the forearms, but Crohn's disease with its multiple symptomatology and relative rarity will be much harder to diagnose and errors are more likely to occur.

There are some tasks that are difficult because of their complexity, and there are a few clearly defined features which contribute to these difficulties. We already mentioned predictability. If every new case is somewhat different from the previous one, it will make the task harder. Another feature refers to the accessibility of the data. Few but the most ardent dermatologists would doubt that the diagnostic problems of psychiatry and immunology are more difficult than those of skin disease. Finally, rare events are more difficult because people have more problems in working in an unfamiliar environment where they have to generate new ideas instead of treading well-worn paths.

These are important concepts for students to grasp. In a teaching hospital they are frequently confronted by difficult diagnostic problems. If they repeatedly see such patients, and come to the wrong diagnosis, they may lose heart and self-confidence. It is important to point out to them that the task is also difficult for the expert and that this is due to the nature of the problem rather than the inadequacy of the clinician.

T: This is a representation of the subject's inferential behaviour. Our intention here is to show how the model may be a useful guide in combining some of the trends we have been following so far. Therefore, we can see now that what was referred to as technique may, in fact, be a representation of the subject's information-processing and decision-making strategies. It measures how he is able to utilize the various decision rules that are available to him so that he will be able to match it with his available knowledge. We have all seen situations where the student is able to recite and correctly weight all the symptoms and signs of heart failure, and where he is even able to detect these features in the patient, and yet he is not able to make a diagnosis. He will be lacking in cognitive control. Work by de Dombal (1979, personal communications) using computer-interacting techniques and knowledge tests has shown that the two parts of the process can be separated so that the cause of the error may be found and remedial measures taken to improve performance.

Systematic errors

A number of systematic errors occur in decision making (Kahneman & Tversky 1973, Payne 1973, Tversky & Kahneman 1974). These are related to the decision maker's biases and are caused by his use of representativeness, availability and anchoring of data as well as the framing of problems when making choices. Errors in the interpretation of the effects of the base rate may result from all these biases and these will therefore require our special attention. These terms need some explanation.

Representativeness

This refers to the choice of alternatives which bear the closest resemblance to some of the essential features of the evidence, ignoring prior probability. This type of error is significant if one alternative is much more likely than the other when judged by prior probability alone. For instance, we may be told that in a lecture theatre of 100 students present, 90 would be from the faculty of arts and there would be 10 medical students. Then, on being told that there is a student present who is neatly dressed with a tie and jacket, many would guess that he was a medical student. According to prior probability, it is much more likely that he was an arts student, but most people tend to judge by preconceived notions of what they regard as the essential features of the evidence. As a result, base rates are ignored and incorrect choices are frequently made. The example where subjects picked a cord tumour rather than multiple sclerosis, in spite of the higher probability of the latter, was given earlier and illustrates this point.

To explore the effect of this bias in clinical decision making, we studied expert and novice clinicians with the use of case vignettes (Balla, Elstein & Gates 1983). In one vignette, diagnostic choices were labelled X and Y to avoid any bias due to preconceived notions of seriousness of disease. In another case, the two alternatives were trigeminal neuralgia or dental pain. Different base rates were given for each choice, but insufficient information was given to make a formal probabilistic judgment. Under these conditions, diagnosis should depend on the prior probability of disease, but the choices were close to 50/50 implying that many subjects ignored base rates. The findings appeared to be consistent with the use of the representativeness heuristic to estimate subjective probability. Judgment was made from resemblance and by paying attention to a strong but mathematically insufficient cue rather than mathematically correct revision of evidence.

Another problem which causes errors with this type of thinking is that people tend to ignore the reliability of the evidence in hand. An example of the '*illusion of validity*' may result when the predictions will fit outcomes, even if these turn out to be incorrect. In the example of a patient who we suspect has multiple sclerosis because some features of the disease are present, clinicians examining his optic discs will frequently describe slight temporal pallor, ignoring the fact that this is an unreliable piece of information, and yet diagnostic confidence will be unduly increased as a result.

Availability

Biases may occur when instances are brought to mind easily and judgment made as a result may be fallacious. Having seen a 'similar case' recently will be one example, or if a patient has some outstanding characteristics, again he will be better remembered. The typical example is having seen a doctor's spouse with this condition, or some colleague, who will be better remembered than the average patient, and thus the evidence will be unduly weighted.

We felt that this heuristic was used by our subjects in a case vignette study where diagnostic alternatives were asthma or cardiac failure (Balla, Elstein & Gates 1983). In contrast to the previously described problems with a rare disease (trigeminal neuralgia) or unnamed conditions as in the *X–Y* case, both asthma and cardiac failure should be well known to most students. It was noted that once more the base rates were ignored by many and the responses could plausibly be explained as being influenced by their recent and salient clinical experience.

Anchoring

After forming an initial judgment, some clinicians may ignore new data. This is the major problem with the early hypothesis formation which is so fundamental to good information processing. There is evidence to show that many people tend to ignore new information even if it is completely contrary to their initial hypothesis. This will then be called 'anchoring' where, in spite of strong trends against the hypothesis, subjects refuse to shift ground.

In another of our case vignette studies we looked at experts and tried to differentiate between the influence of early and late information (Balla 1982). In one vignette cues were given favouring cardiac syncope. The incongruous cue which was given last indicated that cardiac rhythm even during the episodes of disturbed consciousness was normal. Experts and novices frequently ignored this cue and the most likely explanation for this would be the overpowering influence of repeated early cues, all of which pointed in the same direction. Recent computer simulation studies show similar trends underlining the importance of early information (Fox 1980).

The framing of problems

In the chapter on normative theory, we discussed how decision makers would be expected to make choices with the highest expected subjective utility. In contrast, *prospect theory* as developed by Tversky & Kahneman (1981) suggests that real-life decision making is very different and will be significantly affected by the framing of the choice problem. It appears that there are systematic biases whereby if there is a possible gain subjects are risk averse, but if there is a possible loss, they tend to take greater risks. The decision maker overweights low probabilities and underweights higher probabilities so that the choice will be affected by the framing of the problem. This means that the subjective weighting will be affected by what is taken as a neutral reference point. For instance, if one is buying a suit and all the other clothing in the shop window is priced at £30, then a £40 outfit would seem an unreasonable price. Yet, for another item where the average cost was £300, say a refrigerator, an extra £10 would not seem excessive.

If the framing of a question affects clinical decisions in a systematic manner, we should be able to predict which heuristic individuals will use in individual cases. Nisbet & Ross (1980) suggested that much of this could only be done *post hoc*. This was our own finding in the previously mentioned study (Balla, Elstein & Gates 1983) where there were marked inconsistencies in the diagnostic method of each subject. In one case, a subject may rely on prior probability; in another he may use one or other heuristic available. There was no indication that any individual consistently relied either upon prior probability in the absence of other statistical useful information or upon some other criteria. It was therefore difficult to predict in advance which heuristic would be employed. The lack of such systematic biases raised the possibility that medical knowledge is learnt in 'chunks', cue weights are ignored, and that this is one explanation why the diagnostic process is so case-specific.

From the educator's point of view, it must be remembered that students at all grades of experience are prone to these biases and that individual students will be prone to different biases depending on the case. The same thing, of course, goes for the expert. This means that it will not be sufficient to teach a student just to be on the look-out for errors due to one particular heuristic, but that in different situations different biases may occur.

Base rate errors

Mathematically correct diagnostic reasoning depends on accurate probability revision. This involves the correct assessment of base rates so that posterior probabilities can be calculated by combining the effect of base rate information and new evidence. The heuristic biases we described in this chapter showed that we use information according to varied biases and have a tendency to ignore base rates. This was evident in all our studies and there was only slight improvement in the use of prior probability as expertise increased (Balla 1982; Balla, Elstein & Gates 1983). Our perception of what constitutes an accurate assessment of base rates will depend on personal experiences. This was clearly demonstrated in our study of the diagnostic reasoning of gastroenterologists (Balla *et al.* 1983). A group of physicians gave relatively consistent assessments of prior probabilities of various diseases. Similar trends were observed for the group of surgeons studied. When we compared the assessments of the surgeons and physicians there were significant differences between the groups. This is only to be expected as they must have different experiences. Jaundice to a surgeon would most likely mean an impacted gall stone whereas to a physician it would suggest an infection or a reaction to drugs.

There are many other reasons why various groups of individuals perceive these base rates as being different. In our study comparing the use of diagnostic cues by novice students as opposed to their more senior colleagues (Balla, Elstein & Gates 1983), it appeared that students tended to over-estimate those diseases which they regarded as being 'more serious'.

There are basic cognitive problems which affect our perception of base rates and these were extensively studied by Bar-Hillel (1980) and by Tversky & Kahneman (1977). It is likely that at least some of our perception of what constitutes a base rate depends on how we interpret what Tversky and Khaneman referred to as *causal schemata*. They suggest that we may attribute a high probability to a preceding state if we recognize it as being causal in the production of subsequent events. They were able to show that subjects tended to predict events with greater confidence from cause to effect than from effect to cause. They describe an example of predicting height or eye colour in successive generations. The majority of subjects given this task were more confident when predicting from parent to child than from child to parent. Clearly the likelihood of these events was equal.

At this stage we have no clear evidence how this may affect the learning of or the process of clinical diagnosis. We see, however, that in most standard textbooks we are confronted by descriptions of diseases and rarely do we meet a causal explanation which may make it easier for students to appreciate the significance of base rates. For instance, in sections on conditions which give rise to chest pain, we see descriptions of coronary artery disease, pericarditis, oesophagitis and so on. We could speculate that if instead of this method we could describe chest pain as being caused in specific age groups by coronary artery disease rather than pericarditis, or in another age group by muscle strain or oesophagitis, learning may be accelerated.

A knowledge of base rates is especially important when we want to assess the impact of tests on diagnosis. A number of systematic biases have been demonstrated. Gorry, Pauker & Schwartz (1978) showed how normal findings tended to be ignored when assessing new base rates. For instance, if a test is performed to diagnose a certain disease and this test turns out to be positive, then the posterior probability of that disease will be increased. This new posterior probability will then be used as the prior before any further tests are ordered. A negative (or normal) test should have a similar effect in reducing this posterior probability, and yet most clinicians ignore this evidence. We demonstrated opposite trends when looking at the possibility of two diseases co-existing (Balla, Iansek & Elstein 1985). For instance, if a patient has a pre-existing disease such as carcinoma and then develops a new symptom such as a headache, we need to distinguish between this headache being a complicaition of the carcinoma or resulting from the development of a new disease. If a test such as a CT scan is carried out, and this test turns out to be normal, most clinicians would overvalue this result and regard it as strong evidence to exclude a secondary carcinoma as the cause of the headache. On probabilistic grounds the prior probability of this being a secondary is so overwhelming that the negative test result should be ignored. This reveals yet another cognitive bias, where tests are overvalued when they are negative.

All of these findings indicate that clinicians have grave difficulty in appreciating the significance of base rates and there are, therefore, systematic biases in data interpretation. To complicate matters these biases vary according to the task, so that in one situation the information is overvalued whilst in another it is underrated. There is a need for constant watchfulness and a necessity repeatedly to re-evaluate our diagnostic method and to search for biases that may affect our decisions. Self-assessment is difficult because, as shown by Svenson (1981), most of us feel that we are less risky and better decision makers than the average. Until we are able to calibrate ourselves we shall need outside forms of monitoring.

Summary

Four important decision points occur through the diagnostic process (Fig. 8.3).
1 How to evaluate the *data* as being acceptable
2 When to *stop* collecting data
3 When to *reject* hypotheses
4 When to accept the *final* hypothesis.

Data evaluation

This is the part about which we probably know least. Data may be accepted or rejected as being reliable depending on the decision maker's assessment of the patient or on his knowledge of the reliability of the special investigations which he is using. It is probable that incongruities in the whole picture may be especially important in making us realize that the data are unacceptable. The information will then have to be weighted and this will depend on our knowledge of how significant each piece of information is and how it should be integrated and weighted in the situation under consideration.

Students tend to accept data at face value and the concept of the reliability of information needs to be emphasized. Incongruous or negative information is difficult to use and needs a great deal of factual knowledge. Usually only the expert has sufficient funds of knowledge to realize that the information is unacceptable for the diagnosis which is being considered. The weighting of data is usually poorly described in standard texts and if experts disagree, as they frequently do, the student will have difficulties with correct data assessment.

When to stop data collection

When the decision maker, using one of the decision rules available to him, feels that there is enough evidence for the hypothesis under consideration, he may stop data collection. He should also be aware of the sorts of tests available in a particular situation so that he knows whether it is reasonable to pursue the matter further. His

Fig. 8.3. Decision points (D.P.) in diagnostic process.

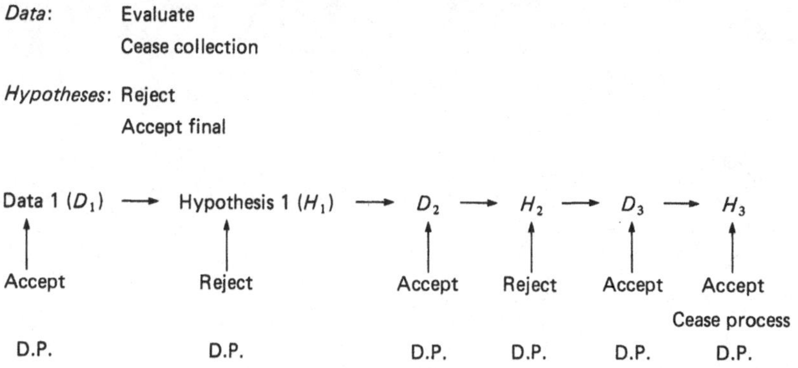

Data: Evaluate
Cease collection

Hypotheses: Reject
Accept final

Data 1 (D_1) ⟶ Hypothesis 1 (H_1) ⟶ D_2 ⟶ H_2 ⟶ D_3 ⟶ H_3

↑   ↑   ↑   ↑   ↑   ↑

Accept   Reject   Accept   Reject   Accept   Accept
                                                           Cease process

D.P.   D.P.   D.P.   D.P.   D.P.   D.P.

assessment of the patient's reliability is necessary to help him decide whether to continue or to stop data collection.

Hypothesis rejection

After taking into account the decision rules available to him, the decision maker may feel that there is enough evidence against the original hypothesis, and so it will be rejected. The main problem here is the one we referred to as anchoring, when in spite of all the evidence people tend to stick to their original hypothesis. It is also important to stress that multiple hypotheses generally need to be entertained from the first stages of the diagnostic process.

Final hypothesis

We saw how the final hypothesis chosen depends on a combination of probability and utility so that the various decision rules used are aimed at finding the most useful and at the same time the most probable diagnosis. We saw how these could be associated with the use of prior probability and an understanding of logic as well as the inherent fallacies of the use of heuristics.

How these decisions are made through the diagnostic process, is something that we shall discuss in the final chapter on the diagnostic process. Before that, we shall look at some of the individual differences between decision makers which may affect this process.

9
Individual differences
❦

We shall attempt here to see if there are consistent differences amongst different kinds of clinicians as far as the diagnostic process is concerned. We saw earlier how performance tends to be case-specific and therefore it is not surprising that relatively little is known about differences in diagnostic technique between different clinicians. We shall, however, see if there are individual characteristics of doctors which will distinguish them as far as the clinical diagnosis is concerned. We shall also see if there are social influences which affect the process.

Individual characteristics
The expert versus the novice

In his work on thinking in chess, de Groot (1965) looked at masters and felt that above all the differences between a master and novice related to extensive knowledge and understanding on the part of the master. He felt that it was 'fecund experience, as distinct from encyclopaedic knowledge' which formed the nucleus of mastership. To be effective for problem solving, knowledge must be combined with experience. This results in an ability to apply the knowledge to individual cases. The expert is able to see the various possibilities of using his available 'know-how' and to see the sequences which could evolve from the situation. In contrast, a novice finds it difficult to relate what he has read in books, or what he has experienced previously, to the present situation. Therefore, de Groot concluded that although there were significant differences in style between individual players, differences in the classes of players were more important.

A study of expert physicists (Larkin *et al.* 1980) demonstrated that experts were faster and more accurate at problem solving than novices. The latter required frequent sub-goals to direct their short-term memory through the problem-solving process. At each stage they had to review progress and search for another sub-goal. The expert would have a clear understanding of the end goal from the earliest stages. It was apparent that not only did experts have a great deal more knowledge than novices, but that this was in a more accessible form. Their findings therefore support the views of de Groot about the importance of the correct structuring of knowledge which is laid down in long-term memory. Gale's (1980) work on the structure of medical knowledge leads to similar conclusions.

It is difficult to find large quantitative studies which show differences between expert and novice diagnosticians. However, Elstein *et al.* (1978) found that experts tended to be more thorough with data collection and formed earlier hypotheses than novice students. The much larger funds of knowledge of the experts were also evident. In a similar study comparing experts and students (Balla & Iansek 1979), we found that experts formed early hypotheses, but that students also tended to do so, in spite of frequent admonitions by their teachers to collect data first and form hypotheses later. The main finding in our study was that experts were good at clarifying their data, in other words in understanding exactly what the patient was saying. Students did this poorly and this may have accounted for many of their diagnostic errors.

In another of our studies comparing students with experts (Balla 1982), students had more difficulty in attaching correct weights to cues than did the experts. In both of these studies, and also in another where the logical thinking of diagnosticians was assessed (Balla 1980*b*), there was clear superiority of knowledge on the part of the expert. Again, it was evident that experts had useful available knowledge which was lacking in students. For instance, when asked to relate symptoms to anatomical areas, even those students who knew the relevant anatomy found it difficult to think of related symptoms, though experts had no problems with this.

Another difference which has significant implications for accurate diagnosis concerns our understanding of prior probability. Not only are experts better in judging cue weights, but there are clear differences in their appreciation of prevalence rates of disease. This was a point demonstrated by Wallsten (1981). We were also able to show that experts are better at appreciating the effect of age and sex on prevalence rates than are students (Balla 1982).

Trying to identify differences in problem solving as a function of expertise, we looked at the logical thinking processes of students in various years of the medical course and compared them with expert clinicians, but could not demonstrate significant differences (Balla 1980*b*). This lack of correlation between logical thinking and ability to solve diagnostic problems was also pointed out by Elstein *et al.* (1978).

A longitudinal study looking at the problem solving abilities of medical students (Neufeld *et al.* 1981) showed little change with increasing expertise. The major difference concerned the content of the early hypotheses. These were more relevant and more likely to be correct in the expert than in the novice. They also proved to be a good predictor of the accuracy of the final diagnosis, so they could make a case to suggest that the content of the first hypothesis will bear a close relationship to the accuracy of the final diagnosis. The work does not extend to clarifying the origin of the first hypotheses, but we may speculate that these are likely to be affected by the clinician's appreciation of prevalence rates and of early critical cues. As both of these increase with expertise and as early hypothesis formation is so important in directing problem-solving activities, these may be valuable leads to follow up in any future studies of the diagnostic process. They further underscore the need to teach the concepts of prior probability and of early critical cues.

It is evident that experts and novices are endowed with similar problem-solving skills. Distinguishing the two, we find that experts have the more detailed and available knowledge which could be equated to de Groot's fecund knowledge.

There are also slight differences in earlier hypothesis formation as well as better data collection and better data clarification by the expert. The expert is also able to attach more accurate weights to the information that he has gathered, especially when it concerns some critical distinguishing cues and a measure of prior probability.

Applying our observations about expert and novice differences to teaching, we see that content rather than process is likely to be teachable. Problem-solving abilities of students need to be developed, but at present there is little experimental work indicating to what extent this helps the mastery of clinical diagnosis. Correct structuring of knowledge is important and, therefore, encouraging students to participate actively in problem solving in the clinic and at the bedside is likely to be helpful. The difficulty in retaining and using 'pre-clinical' knowledge such as anatomy when applied to individual clinical problems, suggests that learning by systems rather than the classically taught individual topics may have some theoretical advantages. This needs to be explored in the future. Our findings concerning the lack of adequate data clarification by students indicates that teachers will need to draw attention to this during history taking with repeated emphasis during introductory courses in clinical medicine.

Teachers have to encourage students to regard prior probability as a 'chunk' comprising age, sex and prevalence rates of diseases under consideration. The major difference between expert and novice concerns knowledge, and in particular it is the kind of knowledge that the expert possesses which is different from that of the novice. Experts know what is important and so they are able to recognize and appreciate the significance of what we called critical cues. Teachers will have to draw the attention of students to these critical cues and the hierarchical structure of information. There should be an increasing emphasis on seeking these cues early in the history-taking and examination process. Students should actively and consciously evaluate their early hypotheses in order to bring them in line with the experts, who not only form early hypotheses but tend to be correct in these early assessments.

Personality

It is difficult to imagine that the clinician's personality would not have any bearing on the process of decision making and information gathering. In spite of this relatively little evidence exists to prove it. Thus, Elstein *et al.* (1978) were not able to show significant and consistent styles correlating with psychological measures of 'dogmatism' and of 'flexibility'. In one study where anaesthetists' judgments were compared, it appeared that their innate 'optimism' or 'pessimism' significantly affected decisions regarding the assessment of patients prior to surgery (Wilson *et al.* 1980).

It is likely that different types of clinicians will adopt different kinds of 'treatment philosophy'; some will tend towards conservatism, but others will be 'interventionist' and more action oriented. These philosophies may then be regarded as guides to their decision making in specific situations (Knafl & Burkett 1975). At present there is no clear understanding of how such philosophies develop. There are suggestions that they may grow through the early postgraduate years of doctors when they are learning specialities and when they have to be socialized into a particular area. For instance, a study of orthopaedic residents showed how they were able to change from a purely theoretical to a clinical orientation. Through these stages they developed increasing confidence in their own judgments. This evolved through stages when they were left to make their own decisions about patients. They were also under pressure to perform well in front of their superiors and their peers. That such personal differences exist and that they may influence patient management has also been demonstrated in the case of asthma sufferers (Staudenmayer & Lefkowitz 1981). According to this study, physicians may be divided into those who appeared interested in the person as a whole and those who were purely disease oriented. The two groups were shown to make different diagnostic and treatment decisions, in keeping with their personal orientation. Little as we know how personality affects decision making, we do know that in any learning process modelling on teachers is a strong influence. Therefore, all of us working in a teaching environment, even when not actively involved in teaching, need to remember how all our actions may profoundly influence the development of inexperienced clinicians who may be watching us or are working under our guidance.

Cognitive style

This was explored by Elstein and colleagues (Tamir *et al.* 1979) in groups of medical students. By cognitive style they referred to the way a person would normally act according to his perception, thinking and problem-solving processes. They defined cognitive preferences as 'modes used by students in dealing with scientific information'. Their findings, though tentative, suggested a high preference for recall and low preference for questioning amongst clinical students, and also that cognitive style may change with experience. This work, as in most other in the field of defining individual differences between decision makers, is at an early stage, but indicates important avenues to be followed. For instance, we as teachers perhaps should encourage and reward a questioning attitude rather than tolerate the passive acceptance of factual information.

Degree of training

Rhee (1972, 1976) and Rhee, Lyons & Payne (1978) in a study of a large number of physicians found that physicians who were boarded tended to make better decisions than those who had no higher qualifications. At the same time, they were able to demonstrate little difference between those who reached no further than the first part of their examinations and those who completed their studies. Older age group physicians relied more on clinical data whilst younger age groups tended to use more laboratory investigations.

Social influences

Eisenberg (1979), surveying social influences on decision making, looked at a number of characteristics apart from the individual features of clinicians. The two that concern us here relate to the doctor's interaction with his profession and any influences that may result from the patient's social background.

Clinician interaction with profession

Eisenberg categorized doctors as being either client dependent or colleague dependent. Those who are client dependent have to live up to the expectations of the patient. They include family doctors or general practitioners. The situation where decisions are made to please patients may occur, and clinicians may also be influenced by patients' demands. We know, for instance, that there are patients who expect X-rays and other laboratory procedures to be performed when they have a complaint and will put pressure on the doctor to comply. In the colleague-dependent category a clinician performs according to the norms expected by his colleagues. There might be a tendency to overdiagnose because of fear of missing a diagnosis. For instance, a specialist physician may have to perform the diagnostic procedures of his field because he knows that this may have been the reason why the patient was referred to him in the first place. If he does not play the game according to the rules, next time the patient may be referred to another physician who is more willing to perform these activities.

At present there is little evidence to show that such differences do exist, but one could visualize them as being important in decision making. These differences are also likely to affect non-medical health professionals, many of whom are dependent on doctors for referral of patients. They may be under pressure to accept the diagnosis offered, especially if the referring source is a specialist. The increasing tendency to work in health teams may change this attitude in the future.

We also know that different specialities will ascribe different labels to the same disease process. This is particularly true when dealing with psychological problems. It was also confirmed by Zola (1963) when he looked at the population of an ear, nose and throat clinic and showed that different groups of doctors attributed different labels to the same patients. An example is the case of vertigo where ear, nose and throat specialists relate the condition to central pathology in the brain stem, whereas the same patient seen by a neurologist would be regarded as having end organ disease in the inner ear.

Working in a team may also affect the decision-making process. For instance, the presence of a psychiatrist amongst a group of physicians may make them more aware of psychiatric problems, and similarly, the recent tendency to have social workers as well as psychologists in a group may make doctors more aware of the importance of social factors when they make their decisions. Problems may also arise when working in an interdisciplinary team when professionals from different background may wish to influence decision making according to their varied perceptions of the situation (Chase, Wright & Ragade 1981).

Although all of these factors are likely to be significant there is to this stage little firm scientific evidence to show that they are import-ant. The most significant finding in the study of Rhee (1972, 1976) and Rhee *et al.* (1978), who looked at a large number of physicians, was that their behaviour was to a very great extent the outcome of the situation in which they were working. The organizational struc-ture of the hospital was more influential than their previous training and experience.

Students being taught by specialists with differing backgrounds may have difficulties in reconciling the varied opinions expressed by their teachers. Diversity of views may have the advantage of encouraging students to 'think for themselves'; confusion may also, however, be the end point. Little or nothing is done in the cur-riculum to accommodate these differences. Eventually, we hope, many students will develop a healthy scepticism towards expert opinion.

Patient characteristics

There is a tendency to ascribe neurotic illnesses more often to women than to men and this has been shown in a number of studies concerning for instance dysmenorrhoea or headache (Lennane & Lennane 1973). There may also be a tendency to ascribe personality disorders more to lower-class patients, but again there is little clear-cut evidence to show exactly what criteria would make a clinician favour a particular decision based on the patient's social background. Doctors may at times be influenced by the patient's ill-ness behaviour (Staudenmayer & Lefkowitz 1981). Those who overplay their symptoms and have difficulty in coping with illness have more diagnostic tests and treatment than those who make less of the same illness. If students are made aware of this it should encourage them to monitor decisions which may be biassed because of patient's social background or behaviour.

From all of this it is clear that we know little about the individual factors which affect the diagnostic process and decision making.

Further studies on the differences between the expert and the novice would be useful and may be expected to result in improved teaching methods.

10

Research methods

❦

This chapter serves as an introduction to the commonly used research methods in the study of the diagnostic process. Throughout the text various references have been made to these methods and here we briefly revise the methodology. Most have implications for medical education and are useful adjuncts to clinical teaching.

Those who are used to dealing with the methods of physical sciences must accept that a study of human behaviour and thinking processes will at times require techniques which are logically distinct from those used for a study of inanimate objects. Of the two main methods available, the first concerns introspection (Radford 1974), when the subject tries to trace some of his thought processes. The second uses various simulation techniques (de Dombal, Horrocks, Staniland & Gill 1971). These revolve around methods for simulating the clinical encounter in such a way that the process can in some respects be standardized and replicated for objective assessment. They include simulation with computers, paper and pencil or with 'actors'. The latter often need the additional aid of video-taping. We shall look briefly at these and refer the reader to more extensive reviews of the relevant literature where appropriate.

Introspection

This involves studying the experiences of a subject during certain moments of thinking. The concept was used by the German School of Denkpsychologie headed by Selz and was more recently popularized by de Groot (1965) in his classic work on chess masters. He studied the thinking processes of chess players using introspective methods. He traced the problem-solving methods of masters and contrasted them with less experienced players.

The introspective method has obvious drawbacks in that once a person starts thinking about his own thought processes, they may be affected by the mere act of self-observation and therefore become unreliable. Often it will be a matter of retrospection rather than introspection. In other words, when a person is asked to retrace his steps he may think differently after he has had time to reflect on the subject and has gained more information than he had at the onset of the process. Deliberate changes from the truth are also likely to occur, but in spite of this we see the technique as giving access to experiences which may otherwise remain unavailable.

Introspection was used by Elstein and colleagues (1978) in their studies on the diagnostic process. They felt that it was reasonably accurate in describing a process, although they suggested that when a subject is asked to attach actual weights to his reasoning there may be less reliability. In our own studies (Balla 1981, 1983; Balla & Iansek 1979) some subjects found it difficult to think aloud, but even without training they had little difficulty in introspection when the interview was replayed on video-tape and when questions were asked at various stages of the process. Some clinicians will be better at introspection than others and after training increasingly useful information can be obtained.

If the researcher is experienced in the field he is studying then he can overcome most of the bias introduced by deliberate actions on the part of the subject. For instance, if a patient is presenting with an initial description of symptoms of diarrhoea and the clinician then asks questions about recent foreign travel, it is likely that he may have in mind exposure to some infection commonly encountered when travelling. If the subject then informs the researcher that at that stage his hypothesis was that the diarrhoea was related to a carcinoma, it would immediately become obvious that his introspection was unreliable.

Introspection has provided many insights into information-gathering and decision-making processes through the diagnostic process, but as it is extremely time consuming and has many pitfalls of questionable reliability and the need for experienced researchers it is likely to be less useful for future research. It is a useful teaching method to ask students to explain their questions and differential diagnosis when seeing a patient at the bedside. Provided it is made clear to them that the procedure is non-threatening, they will often become aware of the errors of their formulations and they may realize that their questions were routine clerical sequences. This recognition may then be followed by new sequences of questions and diagnostic strategies.

Simulation techniques

Among their principles of simulation, de Dombal, Horrocks, Staniland & Gill (1971) suggested that it was important for the simulator to induce behaviour similar to that seen in real life, that the subjects should be able to accept this and should be encouraged to use simulation. It was necessary for simulation to be economical, flexible and realistic.

Simulated patients

Simulated patients were popularized by Barrows (1971) and have gained general acceptance. Such patients are able to produce the closest resemblance to real-life situations and were used successfully by Elstein *et al.* (1978) and also by the author (1981) in various studies of the diagnostic process. They have the advantage that one side of the interaction between doctor and patient can be controlled and it is thus possible to compare the processes of different doctors in situations which can be varied easily by changing the patient. Simulation allows for reproducibility and reliability which is so often lacking in genuine patient encounters with multiple doctors. There are of course problems in that the roles played by the simulators may change to some extent depending on the interaction with the particular doctor. In spite of this, it should be regarded as a powerful tool for studying the diagnostic process under relatively standardized conditions.

Champion & Gibson (1984) have extended the use of simulated patients to teaching and research in the allied health professions. Using an actor simulating multiple neurological problems, they gained ready acceptance by students who related well to the simulated case, overcoming some of their fears of patient encounters in the early clinical years. Their work also proved helpful in developing new models for the functioning of interdisciplinary health teams, a feature of most modern hospitals to which students in all the health professions are exposed. Barrows and others originally used amateur or professional actors, and usually video-taped a patient interview and asked the actor to learn the script from the recording. Most people find it easy to get accustomed to role playing. We have used a colleague and also a trained nurse, which has the advantage of having 'actors' with background medical knowledge so that if necessary ad libbing occurs with ease. It is useful to refresh the actor's mind before each session by replaying the original recording of the real patient. It has been most unusual for doctors or students to have difficulty in accepting the substitute. There has been no indication of deleterious effects on actors of taking on a role apart from the expected irritability and fatigue when multiple sessions have to be performed within a short time (Naftulin & Andrew 1975). In one study students were asked to act as patients in encounters with general practitioners. They found this a useful learning experience showing them how interaction of a consultation was amenable to systematic learning (Markham *et al.* 1979).

Simulated patients can also be used from the educational point of view to simplify complex cases, because the staged manner makes the learning process earlier. This, together with the reduction of anxiety in early clinical encounters, probably constitutes their main educational value. The problem with simulators remains the question of complete standardization of interviews as well as the expense and time involved in such studies.

Video-taping

This is used with increasing frequency (Verby, Davis & Marshall 1979, Verby, Holden & Davis 1979) and is essential to allow review of the various stages of the diagnostic process through the interview. Patients accept video-taping equipment and few will be disturbed by it. Most doctors and students find it easy to adjust, though a few remain tense in the presence of the equipment. The most disturbing feature is the use of excessive lighting and if possible it should be carried out under natural light conditions.

Elstein *et al.* (1978) used film vignettes demonstrating a brief history to a number of different subjects. This results in complete reproducibility avoiding any possible changes in role with different observers. It has the added advantage of saving time and expense when compared with the repeated use of live actors.

Video-taping is a useful teaching method and learners are able to watch themselves objectively and have immediate feedback on their methods. We have used film vignettes in association with slides projected at the same time. On the slides the doctor's thought processes were visualized. For instance, when a patient mentioned complaints of vertigo and double vision, on the screen next to the video-tape there would be a slide projected with a diagram of the brain stem and the words 'brain stem' as floating through the mind of the interviewer. This is consistent with the so-called 'feed forward' method of teaching which is preferable to the frequently used feedback techniques.

In a different context, we also see the increasing use of video-tape teaching replacing clinical demonstrations and textbook learning. Kaufman & Kaufman (1983) found video instructions especially useful in teaching movement disorders which may be difficult to visualize from textbook descriptions. There are a number of distinct advantages in the use of such animated audio-visual material. For instance, in a series of tapes on neurological diagnosis (Balla 1984) we showed brief case vignettes to act as 'triggers' for hypothesis formation. After a suitable pause, these are followed by relevant anatomical and physiological explanations and a reinforcement case. When preparing such tapes, it is essential to make the vignettes brief, otherwise attention sags. A frequent criticism voiced by students concerns the difficulty here in skipping segments, whereas they can quickly flip through the pages of a book. We still have a great deal to learn before we can explore the full potential of video-tapes in research and teaching.

Paper and pencil methods

These are the most commonly used research instruments, though they are of the lowest fidelity as they have the least resemblance to the real-life diagnostic situation. Therefore, any generalizations made from such studies could be questioned. In spite of this they are in general use for testing clinical competence and have also been used by Elstein *et al.* (1978) and others for the study of information processing and decision making through the diagnostic process. One useful way of using these methods is by preparing extremely brief case vignettes to see what sort of decisions a clinician is able to make from the information that is provided. Difficulties arise in choosing the correct wording in such case studies and anyone who is familiar with the problems encountered in setting clear multiple choice questions will immediately understand the identical problem which can arise with compiling such 'thumb nail' sketches. Good case vignettes require input from experts in the relevant clinical area but also need the expertise of psychologists with experience in constructing vignettes. A team approach and repeated revisions as well as pilot testing pay dividends in the long term. In spite of these drawbacks, the relative cheapness and easy availability of paper and pencil methods make them useful research tools. They are particularly useful when studying decision making because of complete control over the information they contain, so that the differential weights of cues can be assessed. Such paper and pencil cases can also be developed into the now popular patient management problems. These are useful educational tools, readily accepted by clinicians (Marquis *et al.* 1984). They can also be developed to measure various parameters of problem-solving ability (Marshall *et al.* 1982).

Computer studies

Computers can simulate various aspects of the diagnostic process. They can be used for research purposes and may also help the development of analytical skills in students. However they are not suitable for all tasks. When a diagnostic problem of some complexity is presented, the clinician is able to think of the multiple disease categories from the patient's vague, ambiguous information and at the same time take into account social as well as personal factors (Barnett 1982). In this type of problem working hypotheses have to be developed and a finite number of alternative routes must be structured from an infinite number of possibilities. Although computers cannot cope with this first stage of picking out a few relevant structures, they may be better than the human brain at dealing with well-defined problems (Blois 1980).

Berliner (1978), using chess simulation, found computers best at search methods along well-defined paths. Humans were better at using and adapting new knowledge but they tended to be more erratic than computers.

Given the proviso that computers are best at dealing with well-defined problem areas in diagnosis, three main methods have been pursued (Rada 1982). These are the formula-based, the flow-chart, and knowledge-based systems.

The *formula-based diagnosis* relies mainly on Bayesian methods. Salamon and colleagues (1976) have shown such techniques to be reliable with a high degree of diagnostic accuracy. In two other studies, de Dombal, Horrocks, Staniland & Guillou (1971) working on abdominal pain and Salamon *et al.* (1976) on neurological disease were able to define the most important criteria for making relevant diagnostic decisions. Thus, although there are considerable problems in obtaining accurate probabilistic information and transferring data from one place to another, these methods can be used to develop a good data base in specific disease categories, and to indicate the most important pieces of information for students to learn.

The *flow-chart based* methods are best for clearly defined paths and well understood problems. They depend on 'if . . . then' decisions.

The most complex methods are the '*knowledge based*' systems. These depend on the flow-chart scheme, but at branches there are multiple possibilities involving many 'if . . . then . . . else' options. The knowledge required to make the correct choice is obtained from experts and thus these are often referred to as 'expert systems'. The problems have to be specific, but the programmes can become extremely complex.

Computer programmes, particularly the ones relying on probabilistic information and knowledge base, may be divided into those which are able to learn and adapt to new knowledge constantly and those which have a fixed knowledge. In spite of the numerous possibilities originally envisaged for computers, clinicians have been slow to accept them. This could be due partly to the complexity of many of the programmes used, but the most likely reason for their failure may be because they have been used the wrong way and their helpful decision-making capacity has been undervalued.

When we look at the potentials and apparent failures of computers as educational tools, we meet similar problems. Arons (1984) describes current uses in science education as having a variable, but limited, impact. Using computers as 'drill' is efficient in saving manpower, and students may be helped in mastering a task which requires repeated trials with immediate feedback. Simulations may also be useful, especially to reinforce previous observations. Students can analyse in detail the concepts involved in the task being simulated. Self-paced courses may be helpful provided that the programmes are not simply books appearing on a screen. The greatest educational potential for computers lies in developing reasoning skills. This can be achieved by the use of programmes consisting of dialogue between user and machine which requires logical reasoning from the student. Similar conclusions were reached in a report to the Association of American Medical Colleges (1983), where it was stressed that computers may be useful for 'conceptualizing and application of scientific knowledge to problems'. The future may also see computers relieving students of some of the incredible load required in memorizing large numbers of facts. A major difficulty stressed in this report concerns the task of teaching the teachers to become computer literate in an era where most students will already be accomplished users. The general conclusion we may draw, well in keeping with our theme in this book, is that the 'logical challenge' presented by computers is much more important than the technology itself (Lincoln & Korpman 1980).

11
The diagnostic process

In this chapter we combine a philosophy of education with a philosophy of science, as applied to learning the process of diagnosis. Our first premise is that learning is most meaningful if it can be related to previous experience (Dewey 1963). If students understand what they are doing, and if they can take the first few steps on their own, they will be able to reflect and then search for the new knowledge that they now see as essential for problem solving. This means that students should not be made to learn multiple features of diseases without preliminary explanations.

An example may help. A group of students with only rudimentary knowledge of chest pain had to work out the cause of the pain in a patient. After asking a few questions from the patient, they reached the limit of their knowledge, but were able to formulate some tentative hypotheses. At the same time, it was obvious to them that they required more factual knowledge. They could see what they needed to learn, that is, they had to find out which of the characteristics of chest pain would distinguish cardiac disease from ulcer pain. They could see that by learning further aspects of the pain, such as its time relationships, they were likely to come up with a reasonable diagnosis. They then wanted to find out about this, which showed that their practical experience was more valuable than being made to study a meaningless list from a textbook.

The next point to be made is that a 'systematic utilization' of the scientific method (Dewey 1963) should help students explore more intelligently and meaningfully. Not only would they be expected to achieve better results with their attempts at diagnosis, but they would also gain more enjoyment from a task they understood.

With experience, thinking often becomes stereotyped and it may be difficult to say anything beyond 'I have had my solutions for a

long time, but I do not yet know how I am to arrive at them'
(Hammond 1980). This should not, however, be an acceptable
form of teaching. We should be able to analyse our processes, and
students should expect explanations based on the scientific method.
As we have stressed throughout, the practising clinician should
derive equal benefits from being able to monitor his behaviour.

We shall now summarize the theories outlined earlier, applying
them in the context of the diagnostic process. Areas where students
are likely to have problems are highlighted so that special emphasis
by teachers may help to avert some common difficulties. This critical analysis of diagnosis should make the learning process more
meaningful.

The first concept students have to grasp is that diagnosis is
usually a matter of making choices amongst alternatives in the face
of uncertainty. These choices will depend on the distinguishing
attributes of the clinical conditions which are being considered as
possible alternative diagnoses. This means that data which distinguish one alternative from another will be most useful in making
the correct choice. There will also be instances where data will be
specific for a particular diagnostic alternative. Therefore, the key to
adequate information gathering and decision making will be an
understanding that the most useful data will have strong distinguishing values or will be strong cues for specific choices. It is
also necessary to combine factual knowledge about diseases with an
understanding of the correct techniques of information processing
and of decision making in individual situations. It follows that
information gathering must be goal oriented, so that heavily
weighted information must be sought from the outset. This can only
be done if early diagnostic hypotheses are formed about alternative
choices. It is impossible to carry out adequate information processing with a completely open mind. Some students find this concept
unacceptable because they feel that unnecessary bias is being
introduced.

Throughout the process, decisions will have to be made at certain
points and wherever possible these decisions should be checked
with logical methods. Even if the decision-making process itself is
not based on strict logical principles, such monitoring is still applic-

able. Finally, it must be understood that diagnostic certainty will never achieve a 100 per cent level of confidence. Students can be taught from the outset that clinicians will always live with some degree of uncertainty. Many remain uncomfortable with this knowledge, and fail to cope for the rest of their lives.

Therefore, choices should be based on considerations of possible utility to the patient. At this stage, we may observe the parallel with what we called the scientific method. Our hypotheses will be tentative, and should lend themselves to being falsified. We should aim for increasing approximations of the truth, but certainty cannot be achieved because there is always room for doubt. To test hypotheses, critical data must be gathered. The hypotheses are formed early, so that data gathering is directed, not inductive. We may reach our conclusions with a combination of probabilistic and utility methods, but the final result should remain open to critical appraisal.

Data gathering
Orientation

The first stage of the diagnostic pathway will be data gathering, and the initial step will be orientation. The patient presents symptoms which have to be sorted out in order to assess the case. The inexperienced clinician may find it difficult to select the most significant information in a patient who has multiple problems. The correct selection of critical cues depends on an understanding of how data are weighted. This is contingent on acquiring encyclopaedic knowledge which includes not only simple lists of clinical features but also an awareness of the weights of information. Most textbooks give lists of symptoms and physical signs when describing diseases. Such a list is unhelpful, unless accompanied by factual information in the context of differential diagnosis. For instance, a patient may complain of recent chest pain and cough. He may have a long history of episodic blurring of vision and poor sleep. The visual symptoms and poor sleep are common in the population, not necessarily signifying gross pathology. Their correct identification will be essential in assessing the patient as a person and will be helpful in determining the sort of approach we may take when forming a relationship with this patient. The recent onset of new symptoms should be discerned as the immediate problem to be dealt with.

How could the student recognize the potential significance of the weight loss as opposed to the lack of immediate concern about blurring of vision? This depends on understanding the prevalence of symptoms in the community. If the prior probability of any person having a particular symptom is high, it is of little help in diagnosis. The presence of this cue may therefore be of little value in hypothesis testing. Weight loss, on the other hand, may have a high correlation with certain diseases, and may be of low prevalence. It should, therefore, alert us to a possible diagnosis. Conversely, its absence may be an even more important criterion in making a specific diagnosis less likely.

Early hypotheses

As soon as these symptoms are singled out for special attention, *early diagnostic hypotheses* should be formed. There is an urgency in recognizing this major aim of the information-gathering process, otherwise data collection will be haphazard and correct decision making will be difficult. One of the major tenets of information processing theory is a need for goal orientation and early hypothesis formation. The choice of the first hypothesis will depend on an evaluation of prior *probability* and of *utility*. Therefore, a grasp of probabilities and of the practical significance of some diagnoses will also have to form an important part of encyclopaedic knowledge. The story of the patient with chest pain and cough may produce hypotheses of chest infection or of malignancy. Occasional blurring of vision and insomnia may suggest that the patient is anxious or depressed, but this is seen as a separate problem. It will influence the management of the primary problem, but at this stage, it must not be confused with it.

Hence, the first stage of orientation is necessary to sort out the various problems of the patient and to lead to early hypotheses, which may then be tested by appropriate questions. We see students who are lost for words after the first few moments of history taking. This is largely caused by their inability to evaluate their early hypotheses.

Data clarification

A clear understanding of what the patient is saying should enable
the clinician to define the specific problems which will require attention. This is the area where the inexperienced tend to make their
gravest errors through the diagnostic process. It is of little use to
know that the patient has chest pain, unless the information is
clarified. Correct data clarification is essential for the proper
weighting of cues. Students need to learn the questions that are helpful in clarifying each presenting symptom. For instance, in the case
of chest pain, the timing of the pain and its relationship to cough
and deep breathing may be relevant. With the cough, it will be significant if there is associated sputum, and if this is blood stained,
smelly or just plain mucus. Encyclopaedic knowledge will have to
include the equivalent of a flow-chart of questions relevant to each
symptom. Most present-day teaching still gives no more than a list
of clinical features, but such charts are available in various fields
and should help data clarification. For instance Hobsley (1980) is
able to list series of questions relevant to surgical problems, and
similar charts may also be useful when dealing with neurological
diseases (Balla 1980a).

Problem solving methods

Following adequate data clarification, stronger hypotheses may be
formed and we shall then be able to choose a problem-solving
method which is suitable for the circumstances. Such problem-
solving methods may vary from the hypothetico-deductive search,
through the heuristic method with the use of algorithms, to that of
simple recognition by one or two critical cues. The method of problem solving will affect the selection of further data. Since different
problems may require different problem solving methods, students
will need to learn which method is suitable for each kind of problem. This addition to encyclopaedic knowledge will result in correct
information-gathering techniques. For instance, most common
neurological symptoms may be dealt with either by the hypothetico-
deductive method or by a heuristic search. Similarly, the patient
who has chest pain and cough may be suitable for the hypothetico-

deductive method. In this method each hypothesis, in this case chest infection or carcinoma, is tested sequentially and a hypothesis testing search is made for each alternative. A history of heavy smoking, weight loss, blood in the sputum and clubbing of the fingers may point towards a carcinoma. An acute febrile illness and cough with mucusy sputum may favour an infectious hypothesis.

There will of course be marked variations in the kind of problem-solving method most suitable for individual clinicians. We are not suggesting that we provide students with strait-jackets for thinking, but we should make them aware of problem-solving methods which are most likely to be suitable for specific clinical situations. Gale & Marsden (1984) identified a number of problem-solving methods used by students and clinicians of varying experience. Their findings show that certain problem-solving approaches can be generalized. Their subjects were not specially trained in problem solving and we may speculate that, given guidelines, most clinicians would find some pathways better than others. This will still leave room for the individual and innovative approach. Gale and Marsden also stress, and we agree, that there is still a need for the traditional routine line of questioning. These questions may, however, be most useful in allowing the clinician thinking time and rapport building, and the pay-off in eliciting diagnostically useful information may be small (Barrows *et al.* 1982).

Cognitive control is achieved by understanding the correct technique that is to be combined with other aspects of knowledge. This will result in a more systematic and effective data gathering and, we hope, in a higher accuracy of diagnosis.

Encyclopaedic knowledge

We see that a great deal of *encyclopaedic knowledge* will be required for this process. In place of learning lists of clinical features, students will have to learn the correct weights of cues, especially those that are of distinguishing value, and those that are highly specific for certain diseases. They will have to associate this with a knowledge of the prior probability of diseases, and of the utility of various diagnoses. All this knowledge will then be related to individual problem-solving methods in order to achieve adequate cognitive control.

The long term and effective *storage* of so much knowledge is difficult and is only useful if it is in an available, *dynamic form*. There is a great deal of evidence to suggest that most long-term stores are not freely available for everyday use by the inexperienced. Frequent and repetitive clinical examples may help to overcome this problem.

We are reminded of a sign in the library: 'Incorrectly shelved books are lost books'. Knowledge must be adequately indexed and stored, otherwise it is of no use. That is why we suggested earlier that when students perceive how the different pieces of information fit together, they are more likely to be able to use this knowledge as the need arises.

The *inherent limitations* of data handling should be emphasized. If only a small amount of data is processed at the same time, it will be possible to concentrate on individual problems, otherwise the system breaks down and information processing will be confused. The need for limiting the amount of information to be obtained is often forgotten by the inexperienced. It is only with an adequate knowledge of the weighting of cues and of the relevant technique in each case that proper data collection can proceed.

Decision making
Reliability of data

One of the difficulties inherent in data collection concerns the *reliability* of the data. Students will need to learn that not only are some data intrinsically more reliable than other, but also that reliability may be affected by the patient and by the expertise of the clinician who obtains the information. Therefore, each piece of information should be assessed from this point of view. The decision when to *accept or reject* is probably the most difficult one to make along the diagnostic pathways. There is little to compensate for experience, but a knowledge of the difficulties inherent in assessing some data helps. For instance, it should be part of encyclopaedic knowledge that a mitral mid-diastolic murmur is difficult to hear and will be missed by many inexperienced observers. The plantar response may also lend itself to different interpretations by different clinicians.

Specificity and sensitivity

Another aspect of data collection concerns *specificity and sensitivity*. There will be situations where even experts disagree, such as for instance, on the implications of the presence or absence of neck stiffness in a child with suspected meningitis. Those who would regard the absence of this physical sign as being sensitive enough to exclude meningitis would opt against a lumbar puncture. Others would claim that even in the absence of such physical findings an infant may have meningitis (Wallace 1979).

More often, however, a satisfactory knowledge of specificity and sensitivity will be helpful in decision making. In our patient with the cough and sputum, for instance, finger clubbing and weight loss would be relatively specific features for a carcinoma as opposed to an acute infectious cause. In the same patient, the occasional blurring of vision and insomnia will be non-specific findings, suggesting an associated anxiety state. In this context we note that the most frequent problem concerns a lack of appreciation of the significance of false positive information.

Termination of data collection

The next decision to be made will concern the *termination* of data collection. this depends on an understanding of the concept of 'diminishing returns'. Data collection should stop when it ceases to be a utility. In some situations, a high degree of accuracy is essential, but in most cases this will not be so. When the risk and expense of obtaining further information outweigh possible advantages to the patient, information processing should be terminated. For instance, in a patient with intermittent claudication of the legs, aortography may be useful, but if surgery is not contemplated in any case then it becomes an unjustifiable risk (MacPherson, James & Bell 1980). At a simpler level, students are generally taught how to distinguish a direct from an indirect inguinal hernia. To this end, most textbooks list certain physical signs. Yet, it appears that no reliable distinctions can be made between the two kinds of hernias (Ralphs *et al.*

1980). It then becomes questionable whether it is useful to teach students to look for such signs when even experts find it difficult to make reliable judgments.

Hypothesis testing

Interwoven with the termination of data collection, the next decision is concerned with the possible *rejection* of hypotheses or at least their careful testing. From this point of view, an understanding of *Bayes' theorem* is helpful. Having learned the significance of prior probability, it will now be necessary to appreciate the influence of new information on this probability.

If the patient with chest pain and cough were an elderly male who was also a heavy smoker, the prior probability of carcinoma of the lung would be very high. If this patient also had weight loss and finger clubbing, there would be no need to change the first hypothesis. If, however, a young woman presented with these symptoms, the original hypothesis would be that of a chest infection. The presence of clubbing and weight loss would then make one think of a chronic infection, such as bronchiectasis. Once this diagnosis was reasonably excluded, alternative hypotheses will need to be entertained, including the possibility of malignancy. Hypothesis testing will therefore have to proceed further than was originally envisaged with limited data.

Common errors that need to be avoided at this stage are those of representativeness and of anchoring. The first, *representativeness*, is due to lack of appreciation of prior probability. It should be part of encyclopaedic knowledge that a young woman with cough and chest pain is unlikely to have a carcinoma of the lung. Strong evidence to the contrary may change our judgment but without this additional information hypotheses should be most significantly affected by prior probability. A lack of appreciation of this concept will result in unnecessary data collection associated with undue risk and expense.

Anchoring is an equally important problem, when, in spite of new evidence to the contrary, the initial hypothesis will not be changed. It is essential to recognize that both the physical examination and the special investigations are extensions of hypothesis testing which commenced at the onset of history taking. Conflicting evidence from these three sources will require re-evaluation both of the early hypotheses and of the new data. The young woman we were discussing may not have an infection, but she may have a malignancy. Alternatively, our observation of the clubbed fingers may be erroneous, or the clubbing may be congenital and thus of little significance.

Final hypothesis

The last decision will relate to the acceptance of the *final hypothesis*. This involves a concern for *utility*. Diagnostic accuracy will never reach a 100 per cent level of certainty. An understanding of decision theory should help to decide whether the risk and expense of further hypothesis testing and data gathering is a lesser problem then the possibility of diagnostic inaccuracy. In the case of a fragile elderly man, we would generally aim for lower accuracy than in a patient who was a previously healthy young person.

Throughout the diagnostic process, an understanding of *decision rules* will be helpful, as these will point the way to finding data of strong distinguishing value and heavily weighted to favour the final hypothesis. Though these rules need not always be based on strict principles of *logic*, the process can be checked by logical methods. It is especially important that the final hypothesis should have some degree of *falsifiability* built into it. This will allow for a revision of the diagnosis as new evidence is accumulated. Unnecessary diagnostic errors are then more likely to be avoided.

In *summary*, we see that diagnosis commences with early hypotheses, probably based on a combination of an understanding of prior probability, early critical cues and utility. Data gathering is then concerned with the acquisition of more critical cues. These will have to be judged reliable and relevant to the hypotheses which are tested. The original cues act as an index to the store of structured knowledge which was acquired through learning. In place of long inductive lists, these structures, include methods of problem solving relevant to the task. Since we know that absolute accuracy cannot be achieved, data collection will cease when further precision is no longer perceived as being a utility.

It is evident that students will need to increase their encyclopaedic knowledge to include correct weighting of data, to understand which data are of distinguishing value, to understand specificity of data and also prior probability of disease, the utility of diagnoses and the problem-solving methods associated with different clinical situations. Students will, however, be able to omit useless knowledge of long lists containing factual information of questionable reliability and of little distinguishing power or specificity for diagnosis.

In conclusion, we shall assert with the great philosopher and educator, Dewey (1983) that 'there is nothing in the inherent nature of habit that prevents intelligent method from becoming itself habitual . . . '.

APPENDIX

Data correlation

Correlations become particularly relevant when we look at serial investigations. If we are to perform more than one test on a patient, we must know to what extent the results are correlated. The fundamental study on this was reported by McNeil *et al.* (1975), who showed that in the investigation of renovascular disease the combination of intravenous pyelograms and renograms added little to the predictive value of a single investigation. We applied similar principles to study the use of visual evoked responses (*VER*) and cerebrospinal fluid (*CSF*) examinations in middle-aged patients presenting with a single spinal cord lesion and suspected of having multiple sclerosis (*MS*), (Iansek & Balla 1984). From literature-derived data we obtained table A1.

If we apply the Bayes equation to our problem, we arrive at the following:

$$P(MS|VER^+) = \frac{(\text{Prior } MS \times TP\ VER)}{(\text{Prior } MS \times TP\ VER) + (FP\ VER \times P\ \text{No } MS)}.$$

Table A1. *Probability estimates in the VER–CSF example*

Data	Probability estimate
P MS	0.33
TP CSF	0.57
FP CSF	0.12
TP VER	0.45
FP VER	0.04

TP refers to true positive and *FP* to false positive cases.

If we now substitute the data from Table A1,

$$P(MS|VER^+) = \frac{(0.33 \times 0.45)}{(0.33 \times 0.45) + (0.67 \times 0.05)}$$

$$= 0.82$$

P*MS*: 33% → 82%.

We see that the revised probability of *MS* is 82 per cent. The common error in these situations is the use of this revised probability estimate of *MS* as a starting point for the calculation. If we were to use this figure, then the revised probability would be 96 per cent, indicating that the two tests combined were superior to a single test for *MS*.

$$P(MS|VER^+ + CSF^+) = \frac{(0.57 \times 0.82)}{(0.57 \times 0.82) + (0.12 \times 0.18)} = 0.96.$$

This, however, is fallacy, in that the *VER* and *CSF* results do not vary independently. Empirical data must be obtained before we can say that the two tests combined are better than a single examination. Table A2 is derived from the literature and our estimates.

It is seen from Table A2 that the true positive rate of *VER* and *CSF* combined in such patients is 0.33 and we estimate the false positive rate to be in the vicinity of 0.04. If we now perform our calculations with these data, the equation appears as follows:

$$P(MS|VER^+ + CSF^+) = \frac{(0.33 \times 0.33)}{(0.33 \times 0.33) + (0.67 \times 0.04)}$$

$$= 0.80$$

P*MS*: 82% →   = 80%.

Clearly, there would be no advantage in performing both *VER* and *CSF* examinations in these patients.

Predictive values of tests

We give an example of the changing predictive value of a test depending on the population studied. The data from the medical literature are summarized in Table A3, and follow from Balla & Elstein (1984) who studied the use of CT scans in head-injured patients.

Putting this in the context of 10 000 head injuries presenting to a Casualty Department we derive Table A4.

Table A2. *Probability estimates of combined VER–CSF results*

	MS^+				MS^-		
	VER^+	VER^-	Total		VER^+	VER^-	Total
CSF^+	0.33	0.24	0.57	CSF^+	0.04	0.08	0.12
CSF^-	0.12	0.31	0.43	CSF^-	0.01	0.87	0.88
Total	0.45	0.55	1.00	Total	0.05	0.95	1.00

Table A3. *Literature-derived data on CT scans in head-injured patients*

Data	Probability estimate
Subdural in head injury	0.003
TP CT in subdural	0.96
FP CT in subdural	0.04
Neuro. abnormal in head injury	0.01
Neuro. abnormal in subdural	0.66

Table A4. *Demonstration of large number of false positives in spite of highly specific test*

	Subdural	No subdural	Total
CT^+	30 × 0.96 = 29	9970 × 0.04 = 399	428
CT^-	1	9571	9572
Total	30	9970	10 000

The total number of subdurals is 30 since 0.003 × 10 000 = 30.

The equations for predictive values appear as follows:

$$PVP = \frac{TP}{TP + FP} = \frac{29}{399 + 29} = 0.07$$

$$PVN = \frac{TN}{TN + FN} = \frac{9571}{9571 + 1} = 0.995.$$

The test has a poor PVP but a very high PVN, reassuring us that the patient does not have a subdural collection if CT is normal. In view of the unacceptably high false positive rate we look at a sub-population of cases. From Table A3 we know that the TP of abnormal neurological signs in the presence of a subdural is 0.66, and that abnormal signs are present in one per cent of the population of head-injured cases presenting to a Casualty Department. This means that there will be 100 cases with abnormal signs in a population of 10 000. From this we derive Table A5.

$$PVP = \frac{20}{100} = 0.2.$$

We conclude that in this sub-population of 100 comprising all those with abnormal signs, there will be 20 subdurals (20 per cent of 100 cases). To calculate the PVP of CT scans in this group we fill in the estimates as in Table A6. (For the present purpose it is

Table A5. *Abnormal neurological signs in 10 000 head-injured cases*

	Subdural	No subdural	Total
Neuro abnormal	30 × 0.66 = 20	80	100
Neuro normal	10	9890	9900
Total	30	9970	10 000

assumed that the *TP* and *TN* rates of CT scans will be the same whether the patient has abnormal neurological signs of not.)

$$PVP = \frac{19}{22} = 0.86.$$

The predictive values for the test have changed significantly and the results will assume a new meaning. The cost of this screening procedure was 10 missed cases in the population without abnormal signs. To find these cases, we will require a different diagnostic method, but that is not our concern here.

Decision trees

The example concerns the use of decision trees in the management of a rare disease where local experience is small. The details of the analysis and the data originate from Iansek, Elstein & Balla (1983), who investigated the debate concerning the treatment of cerebral arteriovenous malformations (AVM).

The first step will be to structure the tree as shown in Fig. A1. The decision node concerns surgery or no surgery. If the surgery branch is taken, then there are three possible outcomes which are denoted as chance events. If no surgery is the branch chosen, then there are two major outcomes, bleed or no bleed, again denoted by a chance node. If there is a bleed, there are three chance outcomes shown as branches of the tree. We next fill in our probability estimates of these outcomes. These were obtained from the medical literature

Table A6. *Scans in 100 cases of head injury with neurological abnormality*

	Subdural	No subdural	Total
CT⁺	20 × 0.96 = 19	80 × 0.04 = 3	22
CT⁻	1	77	78
Total	20	80	100

and when developing such a tree it is best to put these in the format as shown in Table A7.

These probability estimates are then attached to the branches of the tree as in Fig. A2. The probabilities on each node are conditional and therefore add up to 1.0. The probabilities from node to node are unconditional and therefore to obtain the combined probability estimate for each branching we multiply the probabilities. This is referred to as *averaging out*. It represents the total probability estimate for that chance node.

At the terminal branch we also attach a utility value. This is what we subjectively believe to be the utility of that particular outcome. (In the example shown in the figure we attach 0 for immediate death from surgery and 0.5 for death many years later from a bleed. Intact after surgery has the maximum value of 1.0, whilst intact without surgery is taken as 0.9 since the patient will live with the anxiety of a further haemorrhage.) This can also be multiplied in the averaging-out process and so we end up with an expected value of

Fig. A1. Decision tree to show the logical structure sequence of the surgery–no surgery decision in a patient with AVM (arteriovenous malformation).

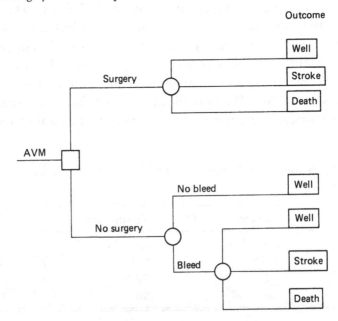

Table A7. *Probability estimates for results of AVM treatment*

Treatment	Mean estimate (%)	
Untreated 20 years results		
Haemorrhage	18	
Sequel: Death		14
Morbidity		20
Intact		66
No harmorrhage	82	
Surgical results (immediate)		
Mortality		10
Morbidity		27
Intact		63

After Ianseck *et al.* 1983.

Fig. A2. Decision tree with probability estimates of surgery–no surgery decision in a patient with AVM (arteriovenous malformation).

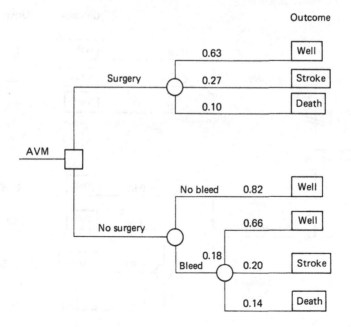

each of the major branches. These are usually shown as circled figures as in Fig. A3. We compare these and decide our preference according to the outcome. We then prune back the unfavourable branches which lead to the decision node. This process, whereby we take the path of our preferred choice to the decision node and eliminate others, is called *folding back*.

On the data available no surgery would be the treatment of choice. If we are able to offer better surgical results than those quoted in the literature, the choice may shift to surgical management. Similarly, a patient's utility assessments could be different from our own, and then we may argue in favour of surgery. It is emphasized that the process does not put the clinician in a straitjacket; on the contrary, it makes our choices clear and logical by making them explicit.

Fig. A3. Decision tree showing utility values and results of folding back in a surgery–no surgery decision in a patient with AVM (arteriovenous malformation).

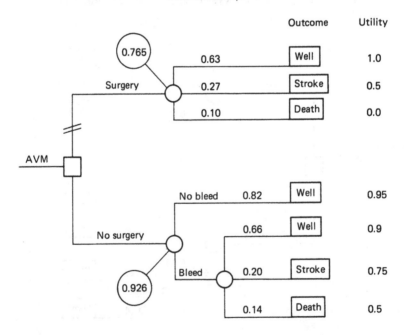

BIBLIOGRAPHY

Anderson, N. H. (1972). Looking for configurality in clinical judgment. *Psychological Bulletin*, 78, 93–102.

Arons, A. B. (1984). Computer-based instructional dialogs in science courses. *Science*, 22, 1051–6.

Association of American Medical Colleges (1983). *Emerging Perspectives on the General Professional Education of the Physician*. Report to AAMC.

Balla, J. I. (1980*a*). *Pathways in Neurological Diagnosis*. Edward Arnold, London.

Balla, J. I. (1980*b*). Logical thinking and the diagnostic process. *Methods of Information in Medicine*, 19, 88–92.

Balla, J. I. (1981). Decision making in a case of multiple sclerosis. *Methods of Information in Medicine*, 20, 16–18.

Balla, J. I. (1982). The use of critical cues and prior probability in decision making. *Methods of Information in Medicine*, 21, 9–14.

Balla, J. I. (1983). Expert decision making in a difficult diagnostic problem. Abstract, Fifth Annual Meeting of the Society for Medical Decision Making, Toronto. *Medical Decision Making*, 3(3), 367.

Balla, J. I. (1984) Introduction to Neurological Diagnosis. Videotape Programmes. Producer, J. Marshall. *Family Medicine Programme*, Jolimont, Victoria.

Balla, J. I. & Elstein, A. S. (1984). Skull X-ray assessment of head injuries: a decision analytic approach. *Methods of Information in Medicine*, 23, 135–8.

Balla, J. I., Elstein, A. S. & Gates, P. (1983). Effects of prevalence and test diagnosticity upon clinical judgment of probability. *Methods of Information in Medicine*, 22, 25–8.

Balla, J. I. & Iansek, R. (1979). The Neurological Diagnostic Process. In *Proceedings of the 5th Asian and Oceanian Congress of Neurology*, ed. G. L. Gamez, Excerpta Medica, Manila.

Balla, J. I., Iansek, R. & Elstein, A. (1985). Bayesian diagnosis in the presence of pre-existing disease. *The Lancet* (in press).

Balla, J. I., Rothert, M., Greenbaum, D. & Black, N. A. (1983). Diagnostic cues in gastroenterology. *Australian and New Zealand Journal of Medicine*, 13, 469–77.

Barnett, G. O. (1982). The computer and clinical judgment. *The New England Journal of Medicine*, 307, 493–4.

Barrows, H. S. (1971). *Simulated Patients*. Charles Thomas, Springfield, Ill.

Barrows, H. S., Norman, G. B., Neufeld, V. R. & Feightner, J. W. (1982). The clinical reasoning of randomly selected physicians in general practice. *Clinical and Investigative Medicine*, 5, 49–55.

Bar-Hillel, M. (1980). The base rate fallacy in probabilistic judgments. *Acta Psychologica*, 44, 211–33.

Beach, B. H. (1975). Expert judgment under uncertainty: Bayesian decision making in realistic settings. *Organizational Behaviour and Human Performance*, 14, 10–59.

Berliner, H. J. (1978). Computer chess. *Nature*, 274, 745–8.

Berwick, D. M., Fineberg, H. V. & Weinstein, M. C. (1981). When doctors meet numbers. *The American Journal of Medicine*, 71, 991–8.

Blois, M. S. (1980). Clinical judgment and computers. *The New England Journal of Medicine*, 303, 192–7.

Borak, J. & Veilleux, S. (1982). Errors in intuitive logic among clinicians. *Social Science and Medicine*, 16, 1939–47.

Braganza, J. M. (1982) Does your patient have pancreatic disease? *Journal of The Royal College of Physicians of London*, 16, 13–22.

Brett, A. S. (1981). Hidden ethical issues in clinical decision analysis. *The New England Journal of Medicine*, 305, 1150–1.

Bushyhead, J. B. & Christensen-Szalanski, J. J. J. (1981). Feedback and the illusion of validity in a medical clinic. *Medical Decision Making*, 1, 115–23.

Campbell, E. J. M. (1976). Basic science, science and medical education. *The Lancet*, 1, 134–6.

Chalmers, A. F. (1976). *What Is This Thing Called Science?* University of Queensland Press, St Lucia, Queensland.

Champion, P. & Gibson, M. (1984). Simulated Patients in the Development of an Interdisciplinary Approach. (In preparation.)

Chase, S., Wright, J. H. & Ragade, R. (1981). Decision making in an interdisciplinary team. *Behavioral Science*, 26, 206–15.

Coles, L. S., Brown, B. W., Engelhard, C., Halpern, J. & Fries, J. R. (1980). Determining the most valuable clinical variables: a stepwise multiple logistic regression program. *Methods of Information in Medicine*, 19, 42–9.

de Dombal, F. T. (1978). Medical diagnosis from a clinical point of view. *Methods of Information in Medicine*, 17, 28–35.

de Dombal, F. T., Horrocks, J. C., Staniland, J. R. & Gill, P. W. (1971). Simulation of clinical diagnosis: a comparative study. *British Medical Journal*, i, 575–7.

de Dombal, F. T., Horrocks, J. C., Staniland, J. R. & Guillou, P. J. (1971). Production of artificial 'case histories' by using a small computer. *British Medical Journal*, i, 578–81.

de Groot, A. D. (1965). *Thought and Choice in Chess*. Mouton, The Hague.

Derouesné, C. & Salamon, R. (1977). Contemporary teaching of neurology. *Medical Education*, 11, 28–31.

Dewey, J. (1963). *Experience and Education*. Collier Books, New York.

Dollery, G. (1978). *The End of an Age of Optimism*. The Nuffield Provincial Hospital Trust, London.

Dudley, H. A. F. (1968). Pay-off, heuristics and pattern recognition in the diagnostic process. *The Lancet*, ii, 723–6.

Dudley, H. A. F. (1982). Axioms in clinical practice and their potential usefulness in education. *Medical Education*, 16, 308–13.

Eisenberg, J. M. (1979). Sociological influences on decision making by clinicians. *Annals of Internal Medicine*, 90, 957–64.

Elstein, A. S. (1981). Educational programs in medical decision making. *Medical Decision Making*, 1, 70–3.

Elstein, A. S., Kagan, N., Shulman, L. S., Jason, H. & Loupe, M. J. (1972). Methods and theory in the study of medical inquiry. *Journal of Medical Education*, 47, 85–92.

Elstein, A. S., Shulman, L. S. & Sprafka, S. A. (1978). *Medical Problem Solving*. Harvard University Press, Cambridge, Mass.

Eraker, S. E. & Sox, H. C. (1981). Assessment of patients' preferences for therapeutic outcomes. *Medical Decision Making*, 1, 29–39.

Fischoff, B., Slovic, P. & Lichtenstein, S. (1980). Knowing what you want: measuring labile values. In *Cognitive Process in Choice and Decision Behaviour*, ed. T. S. Wallsten, Lawrence Erlbaum Ass. Publishers, Hillside, NJ.

Fox, J. (1980). Making decisions under the influence of memory. *Psychological Review*, 87, 190–211.

Gale, J. (1980). *The Diagnostic Thinking Process in Medical Education and Clinical Practice*, London University Institute of Education, Unpublished Ph.D. thesis.

Gale, J. & Marsden, P. (1984). The role of the routine clinical history. *Medical Education*, 18, 96–100.

Gorry, G. A., Pauker, S. G. & Schwartz, W. B. (1978). The diagnostic importance of the normal finding. *New England Journal of Medicine*, 298, 486–9.

Griner, P. F., Mayewski, R. J., Mushlin, A. I. & Greenland, P. (1981). Selection and interpretation of diagnostic tests and procedures. *Annals of Internal Medicine*, 94, 552–93.

Hammond, K. R. (1980). *The Integration of Research in Judgment and Decision Theory*. Center for Research on Judgment Policy, Report 226. University of Colorado, Institute of Behavioural Science.

Hammond, K. R. & Summer, D. A. (1972). Cognitive control. *Psychological Review*, 79, 58–67.

Hampton, J. R., Harrison, M. J. G., Mitchell, J. R. A., Pritchard, J. S. & Seymour, C. (1975). Relative contributions of history-taking, physical examination and laboratory investigation to diagnosis and management of medical outpatients. *British Medical Journal*, i, 486–9.

Havens, L. S. (1978). Taking a history from the difficult patient. *The Lancet*, i, 138–40.

Hedley, A. J. & Pearson, J. C. G. (1981). Audiovisual aids and blood pressure measurement: enhancements to teaching about observer variation. *Journal of Audiovisual Media in Medicine*, 4, 15–19.

Hesse, M. (1974). *The Structure of Scientific Information*. Macmillan, London.

Hilton, P. & Stanton, S. L. (1981). Algorithmic method for assessing urinary incontinence in elderly women. *British Medical Journal*, 282, 940–2.

Hobsley, M. (1980). *Pathways in Surgical Management*. Edward Arnold, London.

Iansek, R. & Balla, J. I. (1984). A decision analytic approach to the role of VER and CSF abnormalities in the management of singular spinal sclerosis. In *Proceedings of the Australian Association of Neurologiest* (in press).

Iansek, R., Elstein, A. S. & Balla, J. I. (1983). Application of decision analysis to management of cerebral arteriovenous malformation. *The Lancet*, i, 1132–6.

Kahneman, D., Slovic, P. & Tversky, A. (1982). *Judgment Under Uncertainty*. Cambridge University Press, Cambridge.

Kahneman, D. & Tversky, S. (1973). On the psychology of prediction. *Psychological Review*, 80, 237–51.

Kassirer, J. P. & Pauker, S. G. (1981). The toss-up. *The New England Journal of Medicine*, 305, 1467–9.

Kaufman, D. M. & Kaufman, R. G. (1983). Usefulness of videotape instruction in an academic department of neurology. *Journal of Medical Education*, 58, 474–8.

Kleinmuntz, B. (1968). Processing of clinical information by man and machine. In *Formal Representation of Human Judgment*, ed. B. Kleinmuntz. John Wiley, New York.

Knafl, K. & Burkett, G. (1975). Professional socialization in a surgical speciality: acquiring medical judgment. *Social Science and Medicine*, 9, 397–404.

Komaroff, A. L. (1979). The variability and inaccuracy of medical data. *Proceedings of the IEEE*, 67, 1196–207.

Koran, L. M. (1975). The reliability of clinical methods, data and judgments. *The New England Journal of Medicine*, 293, 642–6 and 695–701.

Larkin, J., McDermott, J., Simon, D. P. & Simon, H. A. (1980). Expert and novice performance in solving physical problems. *Science*, 208, 1335–42.

Leader (1982). Diagnosis of the doubtful coronary. *The Lancet*, i, 661–2.

Ledley, R. S. & Lusted, L. B.(1959). Reiasoning foundations of medical diagnosis. *Science*, 130, 9–21.

Lennane, K. J. & Lennane, R. J. (1973). Alleged psychogenic disorders in women – a possible manifestation of sexual prejudice. *The New England Journal of Medicine*, 288, 288–92.

Lincoln, T. L. & Korpman, R. A. (1980). Computers, health care, and medical information science. *Science*, 210, 257–63.

Lusted, L. B. (1968). *Introduction to Medical Decision Making*. Charles Thomas, Springfield, Ill.

Macleod, J. (1977). *Davidson's Principles and Practice of Medicine*, 12th edn. Churchill Livingstone, Edinburgh.

McNeil, B. J., Varady, P. D., Burrows, B. A. *et al.* (1975). Measures of clinical efficacy: I. cost-effectiveness in the diagnosis and treatment of hypertensive renovascular disease. *New England Journal of Medicine*, 293, 216–21.

MacPherson, D. C., James, D. C. & Bell, P. R. F. (1980). Is artography abused in lower-limb ischaemia? *The Lancet*, ii, 8082.

Malan, H. (1973). Therapeutic factors in analytically oriented brief psychotherapy. In *Support Innovation and Autonomy*, ed. R. Gosling. Tavistock Publications, London.

Markham, B., Gessner, M., Warburton, S. W. & Sadler, G. (1979). Medical students become patients: a new teaching strategy. *Journal of Medical Education*, 54, 416–18.

Marquis, Y., Chaoulli, J., Bordage, G., Cabot, J. M. & Leclere, H. (1984). Patient-management problems as a learning tool for continuing medical education of general practitioners. *Medical Education*, 18, 117–24.

Marshall, J. R., Fleming, P., Heffernan, M. & Kasch, S. (1982). Pilot study on use of PMPS. *Medical Education*, 16, 365–6.

Medawar, P. B. (1969). *Induction and Intuition in Scientific Thought*. Methuen, London.

Miller, G. A. (1956). The magical number seven, plus or minus two: some limits on our capacity for processing information. *The Psychological Review*, 63, 81–97.

Montgomery, H. & Svenson, O. (1976). On decision rules and information processing strategies for choice among multiattribute alternatives. *Scandinavian Journal of Psychology*, 17, 283–91.

Moraitis, S. (1979). Twenty-one years in family practice. In *Conference of the Australian Medical Students Association*. Melbourne.

Murphy, E. A. (1976). *The Logic of Medicine*. The Johns Hopkins University Press, Baltimore.

Naftulin, D. M. & Andrew, B. J. (1975). The effects of patient simulation on actors. *Journal of Medical Education*, 50, 87–9.

National Health and Medical Research Council (1966). *Report on a National Morbidity Survey*. Canberra.

Neufeld, V. R., Norman, G. R., Feightner, J. W. & Barrows, H. S. (1981). Clinical problem solving by medical students: a cross-sectional and longitudinal analysis. *Medical Education*, 5, 315–22.

Newell, A. & Simon, H. A. (1972). *Human Problem Solving*. Prentice Hall, Englewood Cliffs, NJ.

Nisbet, R. & Ross, L. (1980). *Human Inferences: Strategies and Shortcomings of Social Judgment*. Prentice Hall, Englewood Cliffs, NJ.

Payne, J. W. (1973). Alternative approaches to decision making under risk: moments versus risk dimensions. *Psychological Bulletin*, 80, 439–53.

Peterson, C. R. & Beach, L. R. (1967). Man as an intuitive statistician. *Psychological Bulletin*, 68, 29–46.

Pilowsky, I. & Durbridge, T. C. (1979). The diagnostic utility index, *Medical Education*, 13, 425–7.

Popper, K. R. (1972). *The Logic of Scientific Discovery*. Hutchinson, London.

Popper, K. R. (1976). The logic of the social sciences. In *The Positivist Dispute in German Sociology*, ed. T. W. Adorno *et al*. Heineman, London.

Rada, R. (1982). Automated medical diagnosis – a summary. In *Applications of Computers in Medicine*, ed. Moston D. Schwartz. *IEEE*, Miscellaneous Publications, 188–97.

Radford, J. (1974). Reflections on introspection. *American Psychologist*, **29**, 245–50.

Ralphs, D. N. L., Brain, A. J. L., Grundy, D. J. & Hobsley, M. (1980). How accurately can direct and indirect inguinal hernias be distinguished? *British Medical Journal*, **280**, 1039–40.

Rang, M. (1972). The Ulysses syndrome. *Canadian Medical Association Journal*, **22**, 122–3.

Reiser, S. J. (1978). *Medicine and the Reign of Technology*. Cambridge University Press, New York.

Rhee, S. (1972). Relative importance of physicians' personal and situational characteristics for the quality of patient care. *Journal of Health and Social Behaviour*, **18**, 10–15.

Rhee, S. (1976). Factors determining the quality of physician performance in patient care. *Journal of Health and Social Behaviour*, **14**, 733–50.

Rhee, S., Lyons, T. & Payne, B. (1978). Interrelationships of physician performance, *Medical Care*, **16**, 496–501.

Salamon, R., Bernadet, M., Samson, C., Derouesné, C. & Gremy, F. (1976). Bayesian method applied to decision making in neurology – methodological considerations. *Methods of Information in Medicine*, **15**, 174–9.

Shaw, G. B. (1946). *The Doctor's Dilemma: Preface on Doctors, 1911*. Penguin Books, Harmondsworth.

Simon, H. A. (1957). *Models of Man: Social and Rational*. John Wiley, New York.

Simon, H. A. (1974). How big is a chunk. *Science*, **183**, 482–8.

Slovic, P., Fischhoff, B. & Lichtenstein,S. (1977). Behavioral decision theory. *Annual Review of Psychology*, **28**, 1–39.

Staudenmayer, H. & Lefkowitz, M. S. (1981). Physician patient psychosocial characteristics influencing medical decision making. *Social Science and Medicine*, **15**, 77–81.

Stenhouse, L. (1975). *An Introduction to Curriculum Research and Development*. Heinemann, London.

Stewart, T. R., Joyce, C. R. B. & Lindell, M. K. (1975). New analyses: application of judgment theory to physicians' judgments of drug effects. In *Psychoactive Drugs and Social Judgment: Theory and Research*, ed. K. R. Hammond & C. R. B. Joyce. John Wiley, New York.

Svenson, O. (1974). A note on think aloud protocols obtained during the choice of home. *Reports from the Psychological Laboratories, University of Stockholm*, **421**, 1021.

Svenson, O. (1981). Are we all less risky and more skillful than our fellow drivers? *Acta Psychologica*, **47**, 143–8.

Tamir, P., Schiffman,A., Elstein, A. S., Molidor, J. B. & Krupka, J. W. (1979). Development and exploratory trials of a cognitive preference inventory for medical students. *Medical Education*, **13**, 401–6.

Thorngate, W. (1980). Efficient decision heuristics. *Behavioral Science*, **25**, 219–25.

Tversky, A. (1972). Elimination by aspects: a theory of choice. *Psychological Review*, **79**, 281–99.

Tversky, A. & Kahneman, D. (1974). Judgment under uncertainty: heuristics and biases. *Science*, **185**, 1124–31.

Tversky, A. & Kahneman,D. (1977). Causal schemata in judgment under uncertainty. In *Progress in Social Psychology*, ed. M. Fishbein. Lawrence Erblaum Associates, Hillsdale, NJ.

Tversky, A. & Kahneman,D.(1981). The framing of decisions and the psychology of choice. *Science*, **211**, 453–8.

Verby, J. E., Davis, R. H. & Marshall, R. J. (1979). Television in general practice: the role of a department of medical illustration. *Journal of Audiovisual Media in Medicine*, **2**, 56–8.

Verby, J. E., Holden, P. & Davis, R. H. (1979). Peer review of consultations in primary care: the use of audiovisual recordings. *British Medical Journal*, **i**, 1686–8.

Wallace, J. A. (1979). In *Paediatric Neurology*, F. C. Rose. Blackwell Scientific Publications, Oxford.

Wallsten, T. S. (1981). Physician and medical student bias in evaluating diagnostic information. *Medical Decision Making*, **1**, 145–64.

Weinstein, M. C. & Fineberg, H. V. (1980). *Clinical Decision Analysis*. W. B. Saunders, Philadelphia.

Wilson, M. E., Williams, N. B., Basket, P. J. F., Bennett, J. A. & Skene, A. M. (1980). Assessment of fitness for surgical procedures and the variability of anaesthetists' judgment. *British Medical Journal*, **i**, 509–12.

Wintrobe, M. M. *et al.* (eds) (1980). *Harrison's Principles of Internal Medicine*, 9th edn. McGraw-Hill, New York.

Wortman, P. M.(1972). Medical diagnosis: an information processing approach. *Computers and Biomedical Research*, **5**, 315–28.

Wulff, H. R. (1981a). *Rational Diagnosis and Treatment*, 2nd edn. Blackwell Scientific Publications, Oxford.

Wulff, H. R. (1981b). How to make the best decisions. *Medical Decision Making*, **1**, 277–83.

Zola, I. K. (1963). Problems of communication, diagnosis and patient care: the interplay of patient, physician and clinical organization. *Journal of Medical Education*, **38**, 829–38.

INDEX